Stedman's Medical Transcription Skill Builders

Creating Cardiology Reports

$79.50

Stedman's Medical Transcription Skill Builders

Creating Cardiology Reports

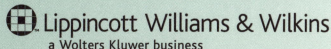 Lippincott Williams & Wilkins
a Wolters Kluwer business
Philadelphia · Baltimore · New York · London
Buenos Aires · Hong Kong · Sydney · Tokyo

Senior Publisher: Julie K. Stegman
Senior Managing Editor: Heather A. Rybacki
Associate Managing Editors: H. Rae Gibbons, Melissa Mathews
Cover Designer: Parkton Art Studio
Typesetter: Maryland Composition
Printer and Binder: Victor Graphics, Inc.

351 West Camden Street
Baltimore, Maryland 21201

530 Walnut Street
Philadelphia, Pennsylvania 19106

Printed in the United States of America

Library of Congress Cataloging-in-Publication Data

Stedman's medical transcription skill builders. Creating cardiology reports. — 1st ed.
    p. cm.
 Includes bibliographical references and index.
 ISBN 0-7817-5531-X (alk. paper)
 1. Cardiology—Terminology. I. Stedman, Thomas Lathrop, 1853–1938. II. Lippincott Williams & Wilkins. III. Title: Medical transcription skill builders. IV. Title: Creating cardiology reports.
RC666.3.S743 2006
616.1'20014—dc22

                                    2006017006

00 01 02 03 04
1 2 3 4 5 6 7 8 9 10

Preface

Over the last twenty years, cardiology transcription has evolved into a complex specialty that extends far beyond the echocardiograms and occasional left heart catheterization that previously dominated the field. This evolution has continually broadened the types of reports that are dictated, which in turn has made cardiology one of the most challenging specialties in the medical transcription profession.

Another issue that is continually gaining momentum in the medical transcription community is the need for strong quality assurance (QA) skills. Many medical transcriptionists perform in a QA role, which involves proofreading and editing reports created by other medical transcriptionists, yet there are limited materials that offer training on how to successfully review, evaluate and edit a report.

In response to these ongoing trends, we are pleased to present the second title in the *Stedman's Medical Transcription Skill Builders* series: *Creating Cardiology Reports*. This unique resource is broken down into three parts: Learning the Terminology, Medical Transcription Practice and Proofreading and Editing Exercises, moving the reader through the basics of cardiology terminology, to actual dictation practice and on to the final step of quality assurance.

By presenting essential, must-have content with a unique blending of the multiple skills needed to successfully complete each phase of medical transcription, we hope that *Stedman's Medical Transcription Skill Builders: Creating Cardiology Reports* will fill a need in your education and practice, and will help you to grow and apply the skills you have learned. As always, we at Stedman's strive to provide you with the resources you need. We welcome your suggestions for improvements, changes and additions—anything that will make this Stedman's product more useful for you. Please don't hesitate to contact us via e-mail at stedmans@lww.com, or visit us online at www.stedmans.com.

How to Use This Workbook

Stedman's Medical Transcription Skill Builders is presented in three parts:

- Learning the Terminology
- Medical Transcription Practice
- Proofreading and Editing Exercises

Each part is designed to give you the skills needed to successfully transcribe and quality check cardiology reports.

LEARNING THE TERMINOLOGY

The opening part of this workbook introduces terms and phrases typically encountered in cardiology reports, including terminology that appears in the Proofreading and Editing Exercises later in the book. Common terms are grouped together, and corresponding report numbers are located next to each term. Definitions, illustrations and other supporting information are also included. Begin by studying this section to learn common terminology associated with the cardiology specialty.

After you have familiarized yourself with each section, put your new-found knowledge to the test by going through the exercises in the Learning the Terminology portion of the *Stedman's Medical Transcription Skill Builders: Creating Cardiology Reports* software program. The practice questions and exercises are specifically designed to help you learn and retain the terminology used in cardiology reports, and the variety of question types and exercises will diversify your studying in order to keep it interesting. See page 1 for more information on how to install and use the *Creating Cardiology Reports* program.

MEDICAL TRANSCRIPTION PRACTICE

Making up the other half of the *Creating Cardiology Reports* software program, the Medical Transcription Practice section delivers 50 audio dictation files covering a variety of cardiology topics, many different dictators and multiple accents and dictating styles. The reports are ordered from the easiest to the most difficult, although your own personal experience and background will ultimately determine the difficulty level for each individual report. Using your computer's audio player and word processing application, listen to the dictation file and transcribe the report. When you have finished transcribing the report, open the corresponding PDF Answer Key. You will find common errors highlighted, along with useful feedback on the various elements and unique challenges found in each report. Each

Answer Key is also provided as a Microsoft Word file, which can be used for further instruction in the classroom or to electronically compare your own transcript to the Answer Key.

Refer to page 67 for more detailed instructions on how to install and use the Medical Transcription Practice section.

PROOFREADING AND EDITING EXERCISES

Proofreading is a necessary skill when working for hospitals/clinics that require reports to be transcribed verbatim. Editing skills are required when working for hospitals/clinics that expect reports to be transcribed as accurately and clearly as possible. Fifty Proofreading and Editing Exercises challenge you to review a collection of cardiology reports for both accuracy and readability. The Answer Keys include comprehensive feedback to explain why changes have been made to the report, along with references on where to locate additional information on grammar, style and usage rules.

REPORT AND TERM INDICES

The two indices in the back of the workbook are designed to help you quickly find information within the text. The Report Index delivers a thorough inventory of the report topics addressed in both the Medical Transcription Practice section and the Proofreading and Editing Exercises, with a cross-reference to each report's location. The Terms Index is an alphabetical listing of the words and phrases from the Learning the Terminology section, along with the page number on which each term can be found.

Acknowledgments

An important part of our editorial process is the involvement of medical language specialists and other health professionals—as advisors, reviewers and/or editors.

We extend special thanks to all of the members of the Editorial Review Board listed on the following page for the many hours they spent sharing their ideas, reviewing pages and reports and helping to make this workbook a reality. We could not have done it without them!

We express particular appreciation to Pati AR Howard, CMT, for her relentless passion and dedication, and to Galen S. Wagner, MD, of Duke University Medical Center, who was considerate enough to share his experience and expertise in cardiology by reviewing each term and definition for accuracy and relevance.

Our sincerest gratitude goes out to everyone who devoted their talents and expertise to assist with content development, especially: Kim Buchanan, CMT, FAAMT; Tamra S. Greco; Xiomara Olazagasti, RHIA, and the team at Orlando Regional Healthcare; Scribe, Inc.; Janet L. Statzer; Marcia C. Stewart; and Kim Watts, CMT, FAAMT.

Finally, we'd like to thank those who worked "behind the scenes" to copyedit, tag and/or QA the content, including Donna Bennett, CMT, FAAMT; Juanita Bryant, CMA-A/C, BVE; Stacy Lehto; Kristi Lukens; Ray Lukens; Kathy Rockel, CMT, FAAMT; and Jenifer F. Walker, MA.

As with all our *Stedman's* publications, this resource incorporates the suggestions and expertise of our many contacts in the medical community. Thanks to all of our advisory board participants, reviewers and editors; AAMT meeting attendees; and others who have written us with requests and comments— keep talking, and we'll keep listening.

REVIEW BOARD MEMBERS

Ann L. Aron, Ed.D.
Professor, Business
Aims Community College, Greeley, CO

Linda A. Bell, M.Ed.
Professor, Medical Terminology and
Transcription, Medical Office Procedures and
Business Communication
Division Chairperson, Business Division
Reading Area Community College, Reading, PA

Donna Bennett, CMT, FAAMT
Medical Transcriptionist, Acute Care
Hospital-Based
AAMT Member

Stephanie Clemens
Medical Transcriptionist, Acute Care
Independent Contractor

Angela Evans, B.S.Ed.
Medical Transcriptionist, Acute Care
Independent Contractor

Tamorah Moore, CMT
**Medical Transcriptionist and Quality
Assurance Mentor**, Acute Care
Webmedx
AAMT Member

Anne Podlesak
Manager, Continuous Quality Improvement
Team
Webmedx

Susan L. Samogala
Lead Medical Transcriptionist, Radiology
University of Pittsburgh Medical Center,
Presbyterian Shadyside

Janet L. Statzer
Medical Transcriptionist, Acute Care
MedQuist

Marcia C. Stewart
Medical Transcriptionist, Acute Care,
Radiology, Cardiology and Orthopaedics
MedQuist
Quality Assurance
Rapid Transcript
AAMT Member

Patti Terrell
Owner
WordMaster Medical Transcription Service,
Owensboro, KY

Bibliography

American Medical Association Manual of Style, 9th ed. Baltimore: Lippincott Williams & Wilkins, 1998.

Anatomical Chart Company. *Anatomy of the Heart* [anatomical chart]. Skokie, IL: Lippincott Williams & Wilkins, 2004.

Billups NF. *American Drug Index 2006, 50th ed.* St. Louis: Facts & Comparisons, 2005.

Cohen BJ. *Memmler's The Human Body in Health and Disease, 10th ed.* Baltimore: Lippincott Williams & Wilkins, 2005.

Cohen BJ. *Study Guide for Memmler's The Human Body in Health and Disease, 10th ed.* Baltimore: Lippincott Williams & Wilkins, 2005.

Green JM, Chiaramida AJ. *12-Lead EKG Confidence: Step-by-Step to Mastery.* Philadelphia: Lippincott Williams & Wilkins, 2003.

Hughs P, ed. *The AAMT Book of Style for Medical Transcription, 2nd ed.* Modesto, CA: American Association for Medical Transcription, 2002.

Katz AM. *Physiology of the Heart, 4th ed.* Philadelphia: Lippincott Williams & Wilkins, 2006.

Lance LL. *Quick Look Drug Book 2006.* Baltimore: Lippincott Williams & Wilkins, 2006.

Medcyclopaedia. Available at: http://www.medcyclopaedia.com/

Medtronic Technical Services. *Pacemaker and ICD Encyclopedia.* January 2004. Available at: http://www.medtronic.com/physician/paceart/MDT_Pacemakerenc_9_Jan2004.pdf

Mosby's Medical, Nursing, & Allied Health Dictionary, 5th ed. St. Louis: Mosby, 1998.

Moses HW, Miller BD, Moulton KP, Schneider JA. *A Practical Guide to Cardiac Pacing, 5th ed.* Philadelphia: Lippincott Williams & Wilkins, 2000.

Rosengarten, MD. Pacemaker Primer [The Online Journal of Cardiology web site]. Available at: http://sprojects.mmi.mcgill.ca/heart/EKGtext/egbindex1.html

RxList: the Internet Drug Index. Available at: http://www.rxlist.com/

Stedman's Abbreviations, Acronyms & Symbols [book on CD-ROM], *3rd ed.* Baltimore: Lippincott Williams & Wilkins, 2004.

Stedman's Cardiovascular & Pulmonary Words, 4th ed. Baltimore: Lippincott Williams & Wilkins, 2004.

Stedman's Medical Dictionary, 28th ed. Baltimore: Lippincott Williams & Wilkins, 2006.

Stedman's Medical Dictionary for the Health Professions and Nursing, 5th ed. Baltimore: Lippincott Williams & Wilkins, 2005.

Stedman's Medical & Surgical Equipment Words, 4th ed. Baltimore: Lippincott Williams & Wilkins, 2004.

Stedman's Pathology & Lab Medicine Words, 4th ed. Baltimore: Lippincott Williams & Wilkins, 2005.

University of California, San Diego Medical Center. Clinical Laboratories page. Available at: http://health.ucsd.edu/labref/default.asp

WebMD. Available at: http://www.webmd.com/

Willis MC. *Medical Terminology: The Language of Health Care, 2nd ed.* Baltimore: Lippincott Williams & Wilkins, 2006.

Willis MC. *Medical Terminology: A Programmed Learning Approach to the Language of Health Care* [textbook and electronic ancillaries]. Baltimore: Lippincott Williams & Wilkins, 2002.

Artist Credits

Cohen BJ. *Medical Terminology, 4th ed.* Philadelphia: Lippincott Williams & Wilkins, 2004. (Figure 2)

Cohen BJ. *Memmler's The Human Body in Health and Disease, 10th ed.* Baltimore: Lippincott Williams & Wilkins, 2005. (Figures 1, 6, 7, 8, 9 and 10)

Katz AM. *Physiology of the Heart, 4th ed.* Philadelphia: Lippincott Williams & Wilkins, 2006. (Figures 11, 14, 19 and 22)

Nettina SM. *The Lippincott Manual of Nursing Practice, 7th ed.* Philadelphia: Lippincott Williams & Wilkins, 2001. (Figure 16)

Nursing Procedures, 4th ed. Ambler, PA: Lippincott Williams & Wilkins, 2004. (Figure 5)

Weber JR, Kelley J. *Health Assessment in Nursing, 2nd ed.* Philadelphia: Lippincott Williams & Wilkins, 2003. (Figure 3)

Willis MC. *Medical Terminology: The Language of Health Care, 2nd ed.* Baltimore: Lippincott Williams & Wilkins, 2006. (Figures 12, 13, 15, 17, 18, 20, 21, 23, 24 and 25)

Willis MC. *Medical Terminology: A Programmed Learning Approach to the Language of Health Care.* Baltimore: Lippincott Williams & Wilkins, 2002. (Figures 4, 26, 27 and 28)

Contents

part 1   Learning the Terminology   1

Learning the Terminology

Understanding the terminology used in the field of cardiology is an integral part of creating accurate cardiology reports. Whether you're new to cardiology transcription, or if you simply need a refresher course, this section provides exposure to many of the terms needed to develop precise medical documents. The corresponding practice CD contains a variety of exercises to assess and reinforce your skills.

The words and phrases in this section are broken down into categories, with similar types of terms grouped together. Irregular plural forms are preceded by *pl.*; synonyms are indicated with the abbreviation *syn*; acceptable variants are marked by *var*. Illustrations have been included to aid in comprehension, where appropriate. Many of the terms are cross-referenced to the reports found in the Proofreading and Editing section of this text (indicated by a report number in the first column) so the term may be reviewed in context, leading to a better understanding of how the term is used.

After studying this section, put your knowledge into practice by going through the Learning the Terminology exercises on the CD-ROM included in the back of this book. Test your comprehension with multiple choice and fill-in-the-blank questions, spelling bee and matching exercises, and even crossword puzzles! Study one category of terms at a time, or select questions from multiple categories. The program also includes a Pronunciation Glossary, which allows you to listen to audio pronunciations for many of the terms encountered in this section of the book.

To install the *Creating Cardiology Reports* program:

1. Close any applications you may have open on your computer.

2. Insert the *Stedman's Medical Transcription Skill Builders: Creating Cardiology Reports* CD into your CD-ROM drive.

3. From the Start menu, select Run.

4. Type **d:\setup.exe** (where the letter **d** represents the letter of your CD-ROM drive), then select OK.

5. Follow the on-screen prompts.

To access the *Stedman's Medical Transcription Skill Builders: Creating Cardiology Reports* terminology review exercises:

1. From the Start menu, select Programs.

2. From the Programs menu, select the Stedman's program group.

3. From the Stedman's program group, select *MT Skill Builders Cardiology*.

4. Choose **Learning the Terminology** from the *MT Skill Builders Cardiology* menu screen.

A comprehensive Help File is included to help you navigate the program.

Once you have learned the terminology used in cardiology reports, move on to Part 2: Medical Transcription Practice and begin transcribing actual physician dictation. Refer to p. 67 for more information on how to use the Medical Transcription Practice section.

CARDIOLOGY TERMINOLOGY

Common Prefixes, Suffixes and Combining Forms

Term	Definition
a-	without, not
-al	pertaining to
angi/o	vessel
ante-	before
anti-	against, opposed to
aort/o	aorta
-ar, -ary	pertaining to
arteri/o	artery
ather/o	fatty, paste, soft
-ation	process
atri/o	atrium
bi-	two
-brady, brady-	slow
cardi/o	heart
coagul/o	to clot
cor-	heart
coron/o	crown, circle
de-	from, down, not
dia-	across, through
dys-	painful, difficult, faulty
echo-	a reverberating sound; the acoustic signal on ultrasonography
-ectasia, -ectasis	dilation, expansion
-ectomy	removal, surgical removal
-emia	blood condition
endo-	inner, within
epi-	outer, upon
erythr/o	red
extra-	outside
-genesis	production, beginning

Term	Definition
-gram	a recording
-graph	an instrument used for recording
-graphy	the process of recording, writing or describing
hem/o	blood
hol/o	whole, entire, complete
hyper-	above, excessive
hypo-	below, decreased
-ia	condition of
-ic	pertaining to
infra-	below, under
intra-	within
-ist	one who specializes in
-itis	inflammation
-ium	lining, membrane
kinesi/o	movement
-logy	study of
mamm/o	breast
-meter	an instrument for measuring
-metry	the process of measuring
mono-	one
morph/o	form, shape, structure
my/o, myo-	muscle
-oma	mass or tumor
-osis	condition of
-ous	pertaining to
-pathy	disease
pector/o	chest
ped/o	foot; child
peri-	around, surrounding
phleb/o	vein
-plasty	surgical repair or reconstruction
-plegia	paralysis

Term	Definition
pleur/a, pleur/o	pleural cavity, rib, side
-pnea	breathing
post-	after; behind
pre-	before
pulm/o, pulmon/o	lung
retro-	behind, backward
scler/o	hardening
-scope	an instrument for examining
semi-	half
-spasm	an involuntary contraction
sphygm/o	pulse
-stasis	stop, stand
sten/o	narrow
stern/o	sternum, breastbone
steth/o	chest
sub-	under, below
supra-	above, excessive
tachy-	fast
tel/e, tel/o	distance, other end
thorac/o, thoracic/o	chest, thoracic cavity
thromb/o	clot
-tion	process
trans-	across; through
tri-	three
trop/o	a turning
uni-	one
valv/o, valvul/o	valve
varic/o	a twisted, swollen vein
vas/o, vascul/o	blood vessel
ven/i, ven/o	vein
ventricul/o	ventricle, belly, pouch
-y	process of, condition

General Cardiovascular Terms

Report #	Term	Definition
	adventitious	Arising from an external source or occurring in an unusual place or manner.
	afebrile	Without fever, denoting apyrexia; having a normal body temperature.
23	akinetic	Pertaining to the absence or loss of power in voluntary movement.
	ambulating; ambulatory	Walking about or able to walk about; denoting a patient who is not confined to a bed as a result of disease or surgery.
35	anastomosis, *pl.* anastomoses	An operative union of two structures (e.g., vessels, ureters, nerves).
	aneurysmal	Relating to a widening or bulging of the wall of the heart, the aorta or an artery caused by congenital defect or acquired weakness.
1	antegrade	In the direction of normal movement, as in blood flow or peristalsis. Opposite of retrograde.
48	anterolateral	In front and away from the middle line.
	anticoagulant	An agent that prevents clotting.
10	anticoagulate; anticoagulated; anticoagulation	To prevent clotting or curdling.
	antihypertensives	A category of drugs used for treatment of high blood pressure.
	arrest	A stoppage; interference with the regular course of performance of the heart's function.
	artifact	Anything in a graphic record that is caused by the technique used and not reflecting the original specimen or experiment; sometimes called "noise."
8	asymptomatic	Without symptoms; producing no symptoms.
	atelectasis	A decrease or loss of air in all or part of the lung, with resulting loss of lung volume.
17	atherosclerotic; atherosclerotic changes	Pertaining to a degenerative condition of the arteries with thickening of the inner lining due to a build-up of plaque, loss of elasticity, and susceptibility to rupture; seen most often in the aged or smokers.
20	atmosphere	A unit of air pressure.
11	atraumatic	Not relating to, caused by or affected by trauma.
7	atrial	Pertaining to the two upper chambers of the heart.
12	atypical	Not usual or typical; not corresponding to the normal form or type.

Report #	Term	Definition
9	baseline (ECG, heart rate, blood pressure)	The number, measurement or calculation considered to be normal for a particular patient and against which subsequent measurements are compared. In some diagnostic studies, the baseline may be determined by readings obtained from a patient during a period of stability.
8	bifurcate; bifurcating; bifurcation	To fork; to divide into two branches.
28	biphasic	Two separate and distinct phases.
	blunt dissection	In an operation, to separate the different structures along natural lines by dividing the connective tissue framework without cutting.
26	bolus	A single, relatively large quantity of a substance, usually one intended for therapeutic use, such as a bolus dose of a drug injected intravenously.
4	bruit	An auscultatory sound, produced in a blood vessel, usually arterial.
1	bypass	*(verb)* To create new flow from one structure to another through a diversionary channel.
6	calcify; calcified; calcification	The process in which tissue or noncellular material in the body hardens as the result of precipitates or larger deposits of insoluble salts of calcium, as in calcified coronary artery plaque.
8	cannulate; cannulated; cannulation, *var.* cannulization	Insertion of a cannula.
2	cardiac	Pertaining to the heart.
40	cardiac output	The product of heart rate and heart stroke volume, measured in liters per minute; the amount of blood that is pumped by the heart in 1 minute.
27	cardioplegia	Paralysis of the heart; an elective temporary cessation of cardiac activity by injection of chemicals, selective hypothermia or electrical stimuli and used to perform surgery on the heart.
2	catheterization; catheterize	To pass a catheter.
	cauterize	An agent or device used for scarring, burning or cutting the skin or other tissues by means of heat, cold, electric current, ultrasound or caustic chemicals.
9	chronic	In reference to a health-related state, lasting a long time.
	chronic obstructive pulmonary disease (COPD)	A general term used for those diseases with permanent or temporary narrowing of bronchi, in which forced expiratory flow is slowed, especially when no etiologic or other more specific term can be applied. Usually in reference to bronchitis or emphysema.

Report #	Term	Definition
30	commissure	The union of two anatomical parts to form a corner.
6	concentric	Having a common center, such that two or more spheres, circles or segments of circles are inside one another.
40	contractility	The ability or property of a substance, especially of muscle, to shorten, or become smaller, or develop increased tension.
8	COPD	Abbreviation for chronic obstructive pulmonary disease.
44	crossclamp, *var.* cross-clamp	A technique of compression using a cruciate or cross formation.
43	damping	Bringing a mechanism to rest with minimal oscillation.
	débridement	Removal of foreign materials, necrotic matter and devitalized tissue from a wound or burn.
15	defibrillator	Any electrical agent or measure that arrests fibrillation of the ventricular muscle and restores the normal beat.
4	diaphoresis	The excretion of fluid by the sweat glands of the skin. *Syn:* perspiration
6	diastole; diastolic	The period in the cardiac cycle when blood enters the relaxed ventricles from the atria; the second measurement of blood pressure. See Figure 1.
	dilation	The act of stretching or enlarging an opening or the lumens of a hollow structure (e.g., an artery). *Syn:* dilatation
	dilatation	*Syn:* dilation
20	dissection	In an operation, the act of separating the different structures along natural lines by dividing the connective tissue framework.

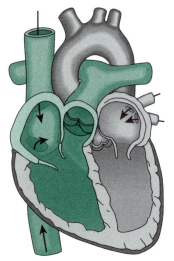

Diastole
Atria fill with blood, which begins to flow into ventricles as soon as their walls relax.

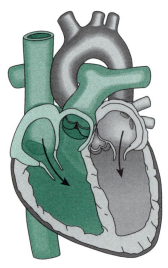

Atrial systole
Contraction of atria pumps blood into the ventricles.

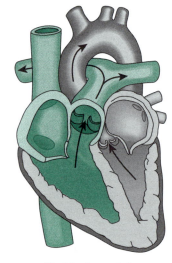

Ventricular systole
Contraction of ventricles pumps blood into aorta and pulmonary arteries.

FIGURE 1. The cardiac cycle.

Report #	Term	Definition
	double product	A measure of heart workload determined by multiplying systolic blood pressure with the heart frequency.
26	dual chamber	Referring to the two chambers of the heart; usually refers to pacemaker leads placed in both the right atrium and the right ventricle (e.g., dual-chamber ICD, dual-chamber device).
4	dyspnea	Shortness of breath, usually associated with disease of the heart or lungs.
5	ectasia	Dilation of a tubular structure.
48	ectatic	Pertaining to the dilation of a tubular structure.
6	effusion	The increase of fluid in a space into the tissues or a cavity.
6	ejection fraction	The fraction of the blood contained in the ventricle at the end of diastole that is expelled during its contraction.
9	embolus, *pl.* emboli	A plug composed of a detached thrombus or vegetation, mass of bacteria or other foreign body that moves from elsewhere to occlude a blood vessel; do not confuse with thrombus, which is formed from blood constituents.
16	emphysema	Pulmonary disease characterized by dilation and destruction of the alveoli.
21	end-diastolic pressure	The intracardiac pressure at the end of diastole, immediately before the next systole.
4	epigastric	Pertaining to the area above the stomach.
	erythema	Redness due to capillary dilation.
	ethyl alcohol	Ethanol made from carbohydrates by fermentation and synthetically from ethylene or acetylene. Medicinally, it is used externally as a rubefacient, coolant and disinfectant, and internally as an analgesic, stomachic and sedative.
	etiology	The science of causes, causality; in common usage, cause.
	exsanguinate	To remove or withdraw circulating blood; to make bloodless.
28	fascia, *pl.* fasciae, fascias	A sheet of fibrous tissue that envelops the body beneath the skin; it also encloses muscles and groups of muscles, and separates their several layers or groups.
44	flush; flushed	A transient erythema due to heat, exertion, stress or disease.
15	frequency	In reference to the heart, the number of heartbeats per minute.
4	gallop	An abnormal third or fourth heart sound being heard in addition to the first and second sounds; sometimes indicative of serious disease.
	gastric angiodysplasia	A degenerative or congenital structural abnormality of the normally distributed vasculature of the stomach.
15	gastrointestinal (GI) bleeding	Bleeding from the stomach or intestinal tract.

Report #	Term	Definition
	gentle massage technique	A method used during open heart surgery to remove air from the left ventricle.
39	global	The complete, generalized, overall or total aspect.
21	gradient	Rate of change of temperature, pressure, magnetic field or other variable as a function of distance, time or other scale.
	hemangioma	A congenital anomaly in which proliferation of blood vessels leads to a mass that resembles a neoplasm; it can occur anywhere in the body.
4	hematuria	The presence of blood or red blood cells in the urine.
12	hemodynamic	Relating to the physical aspects of the blood circulation.
25	hemostasis; hemostatic	The arrest of bleeding; the arrest of circulation in a part.
44	heparinize; heparinization	To perform therapeutic administration of heparin.
	hypertensor	*Syn:* pressor
	hypocoagulable	Decreased ability of blood to coagulate or clot.
	hypodense focus, *pl.* hypodense foci	An area of less than normal density.
43	hypokinesis	In relation to cardiology, diminished systolic inward movement of the myocardium.
43	inferior aspect	Situated below or directed downward (e.g., LV wall positioned on the diaphragm).
27	infusion	The introduction of fluid other than blood (e.g., saline solution) into a vein.
	inotrope	A substance that alters the force of muscular contractility.
44	inotropic support	Assisting the contractility of muscular tissue.
8	insufficiency	Lack of completeness of function or power.
4	intermittent	Marked by intervals of complete quietude between two periods of activity.
	intima	Innermost.
	intimal	Relating to the intima or inner coat of a vessel.
	intraatrial	Within the atria.
26	intracardiac	Within the heart.
	intracavitary	Within a (heart) cavity.
8	intravenous (IV)	Within a vein or veins.
	IV	Abbreviation for intravenous.

Report #	Term	Definition
	jugular	Relating to the jugular veins.
44	lumen	The space in the interior of a tubular structure such as an artery or the intestine.
29	luminal	Pertaining to the space in the interior of a tubular structure, such as an artery.
	MET, *pl.* METs	Abbreviation for metabolic equivalent.
	metabolic equivalent (MET)	The oxygen cost of energy expenditure measured during supine rest.
4	murmur	A sound, like that made by a somewhat forcible expiration with the mouth open, heard on auscultation of the heart. When heard over blood vessels, it is termed bruit.
	myocardial	Referring to the middle layer of the heart.
	nonocclusive	Not closing or blocking a passageway.
	oblique caudal view	In radiography, a projection from the direction of the lower (caudal) part of the body that is neither frontal nor lateral, but slanting.
	oblique cranial view	In radiography, a projection from the direction of the head that is neither frontal nor lateral, but slanting.
43	oblique view	In radiography, a projection that is neither frontal nor lateral, but slanting.
1	occlude; occlusion	To close (e.g., coronary occlusion).
4	orthopnea	Discomfort in breathing that is brought on or aggravated by lying flat.
	output	See: cardiac output
8	pacemaker	Biologically, any rhythmic center that establishes a pace of activity; an artificial regulator of rate activity. When referring to an artificial regulator, it can also be called a pulse generator. See Figure 2. *Syn:* pulse generator
	paroxysmal	Pertaining to the sudden onset of a symptom or disease.
	paroxysmal nocturnal dyspnea	A sudden onset of difficultly in breathing that occurs at night, several hours after assuming a recumbent position.
1	patent	Open or exposed.
	PCP	Abbreviation for primary care physician.
	perfusion	The flow of blood.
24	pericardiac, *var.* pericardial	Surrounding the heart; relating to the pericardium.
	pericardial friction sound	*Syn:* pericardial rub

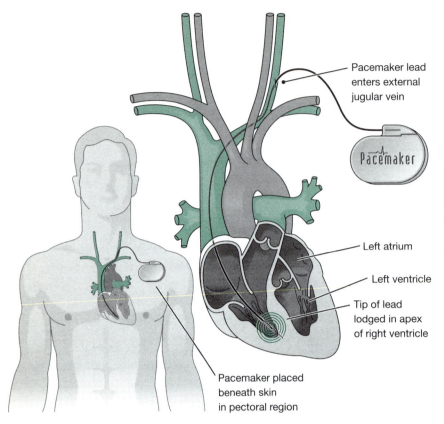

FIGURE 2. Placement of a pacemaker. The lead is placed in an atrium or ventricle (usually on the right side). A dual-chamber pacemaker has a lead in both chambers.

Report #	Term	Definition
	pericardial rub	A to-and-fro grating, rasping or, rarely, creaking sound heard over the heart in some cases of pericarditis, due to rubbing of the inflamed pericardial surfaces as the heart contracts and relaxes. *Syn:* pericardial friction sound
	perspiration	*Syn:* diaphoresis
5	plaque	Fatty material that deposits in vessel linings.
30	pleura, *pl.* pleurae	The serous membrane enveloping the lungs and lining the walls of the pleural cavity.
	pleural effusion	Increased fluid in the pleural space.
13	pressor	Producing increased blood pressure. *Syn:* hypertensor
	primary care physician (PCP)	A medical doctor who provides a basic level of health care.
2	proximal; proximal portion	Nearest to the point of origin.
	pulmonary fibrosis	A connective tissue disease of the lungs.
	purpuric patches	A condition characterized by hemorrhaging into the skin.
44	reapproximate	To put back together; to close.
6	regurgitation	A backward flow, as of blood through an incompetent valve of the heart.

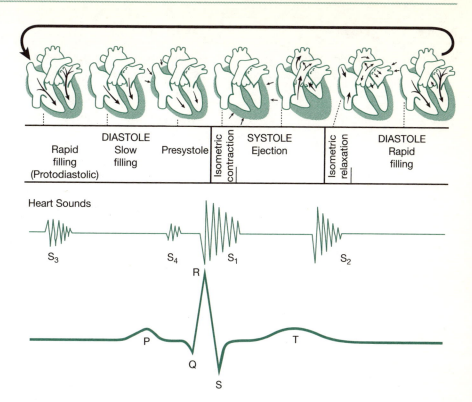

FIGURE 3. Electrocardiogram. The cardiac cycle consists of filling and ejection. Heart sounds S_2, S_3 and S_4 are associated with diastole, while S_1 is associated with systole. The electrical activity of the heart is measured throughout diastole and systole by electrocardiography.

Report #	Term	Definition
	residual lesion	That which remains after removal of a substance.
26	retrograde	Moving backward; the opposite of antegrade.
4	S_1, S_2, S_3, S_4	Symbols for first, second, third and fourth heart sounds; may be written as S1, S2, S3 and S4 in patient records. See Figure 3.
	spurious	False; not genuine.
2	stenosis; focal stenosis	A narrowing or stricture of any canal or localized area.
2	stent; stenting	A small tube inserted into a vessel to keep it open. See Figure 4.
2	subsequent	Later in time or order.
3	supine	Denoting the body when lying face upward.
8	symptomatic	Pertaining to the presence of symptoms.

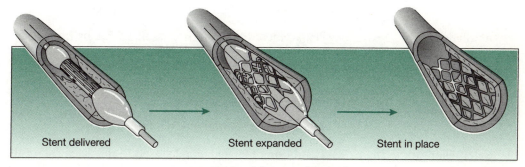

FIGURE 4. Intravascular stent.

Report #	Term	Definition
6, 41	systole; systolic	Pertaining to the period in the cardiac cycle when the heart is contracting and blood is ejected from the ventricles. See Figure 1.
5	takeoff	The beginning or point of origin, as in the takeoff of an artery branch.
14	target	A value fixed as the goal or point of examination, as in a target heart rate.
	telemetry	The transmission of cardiac signals (derived from electricity or pressure) to a receiving location where they are displayed for monitoring.
3, 6	thrombus, *pl.* thrombi	A stationary blood clot formed from blood constituents; do not confuse with embolus, which is formed from foreign materials.
	tortuous	Having many curves; full of turns and twists.
	transect; transection	To cut across.
25	transesophageal	Pertaining to across or through the esophagus.
29	transluminal	Pertaining to across or through the lumen of a vessel.
26	transvenous	Pertaining to across or through a vein.
43	trifurcate; trifurcation	To divide into three branches.
	valvule	A valve, especially a small one.
6	valvular	Pertaining to a valve.
31	velocity	Rate of movement, specifically, distance traveled or quantity converted per unit time in a given direction.
17	vegetation	Specifically, a clot composed largely of fused blood platelets, fibrin and sometimes microorganisms, which adhere to a diseased heart orifice or valve; often initiated by infection of the structures involved.
9	venous stasis	Congestion and slowing of circulation in the veins due to blockage by either obstruction or high pressure in the venous system, seen most frequently in the feet and legs.
2	vent	An opening into a cavity or canal, especially one through which the contents of such a cavity are discharged.
	ventilation	Replacement of air or other gas in a space by fresh air or gas.
43	ventricularization	Transformation of an atrial phenomenon to simulate a ventricular one, especially of the atrial (or venous) pulse tracing in tricuspid regurgitation.
15	vertigo	A sensation of spinning or whirling motion.
	watermelon stomach	Condition of dilated blood vessels in the distal end of the stomach.

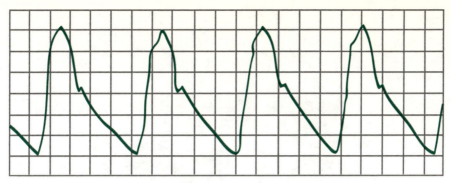

FIGURE 5. Normal arterial waveform.

Report #	Term	Definition
	waveform	The representation of a wave on a graph (e.g., an arterial pressure or displacement wave; or the pacemaker pulse as demonstrated on an oscilloscope under a specified load). See Figure 5.

Anatomical Terminology

Cardiac anatomy

Report #	Term	Definition
	anteroseptal segment of the apex	Section of the anterior septal wall at the bottom point of the heart.
	aortic cusp	One of the three fibrous semilunar leaflets or valvules of the aortic valve between the left ventricle and the ascending aorta.
6	aortic valve	The valve between the left ventricle and the ascending aorta, consisting of three fibrous semilunar cusps (valvules or leaflets). See Figure 6. *Syn:* trileaflet aortic valve
	apex	The cone-shaped area of the heart formed by the joining of the left and right ventricles. See Figure 6. *Syn:* ventricular apex
17	atrial appendage	A small conical pouch projecting from the upper anterior portion of each atrium of the heart, increasing the atrial volume slightly. *Syn:* auricle (of atrium)
	atrial septum	*Syn:* interatrial septum
	atrioventricular groove	A groove on the outer surface of the heart marking the division between the atria and the ventricles. *Syn:* coronary sulcus
11, 17	atrium, *pl.* atria	One of the two upper chambers of the heart. See Figure 6.
	auricle (of atrium)	*Syn:* atrial appendage

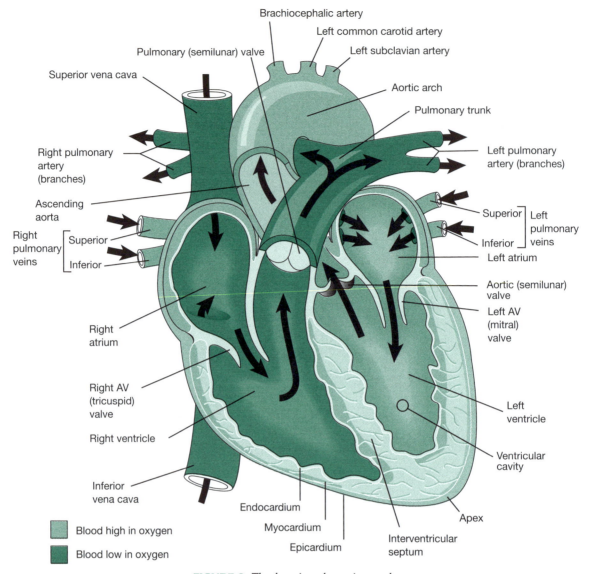

FIGURE 6. The heart and great vessels.

Report #	Term	Definition
26	AV node	A bundle of electroconductive fibers dividing into right and left bundles.
	bicuspid valve	*Syn:* mitral valve
26	bundle of His	Specialized cardiac fibers that divide into two branches.
6	chamber	A compartment or enclosed space, referring to the two atria and two ventricles of the heart.
17	chorda, *pl.* chordae	A tendinous or cord-like structure. See Figure 7.
	chordae tendineae	The tendinous strands running from the papillary muscles to the leaflets of the atrioventricular valves.
	coronary sulcus	*Syn:* atrioventricular groove
6	cusp	A leaflet of one of the heart's valves. See Figure 7.

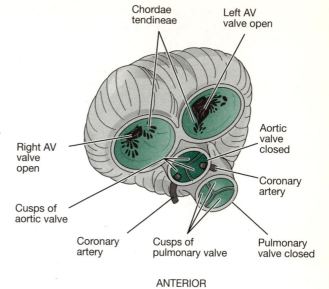

POSTERIOR

Chordae tendineae

Left AV valve open

Aortic valve closed

Coronary artery

Right AV valve open

Cusps of aortic valve

Coronary artery

Cusps of pulmonary valve

Pulmonary valve closed

ANTERIOR

FIGURE 7. The valves of the heart shown during diastole.

Report #	Term	Definition
	endocardium	The innermost tunic of the heart.
	epicardium	The visceral layer of serous pericardium.
22	inferolateral	Involving the inferior and lateral surfaces of the left ventricle and producing indicative changes in the electrocardiogram in leads II, III, aVF, V_1 and V_2.
17	interatrial septum	The wall between the atria of the heart; when transcribing, be careful to type as interatrial and not intraatrial.
	internodal pathway	Specialized cardiac fibers in the walls of the atrium.
23	interventricular	Between the ventricles.
	interventricular septum	The wall between the ventricles of the heart; when transcribing, be careful to use inter- and not intra-. See Figure 6. *Syn:* ventricular septum
31	intraventricular	Within a (heart) ventricle.
17	leaflet	A thin flattened object or structure associated with the heart valves.
2	left ventricle (LV)	The lower chamber of the left side of the heart that receives the arterial blood from the left atrium and drives it by the contraction of its walls into the aorta. See Figure 6.
4	LV	Abbreviation for left ventricle.
17	mitral valve	The valve closing the orifice between the left atrium and left ventricle of the heart; its two cusps are called anterior and posterior. See Figure 6. *Syn:* bicuspid valve

Report #	Term	Definition
	myocardium, *pl.* myocardia	The middle layer of the heart; the cardiac muscle. See Figure 6.
31	papillary muscle	One of the group of myocardial bundles that originate at the endocardium and terminate in the chordae tendineae and attach to the cusps of the atrioventricular valves; each ventricle has an anterior and a posterior papillary muscle. See Figure 8.
27	pericardium, *pl.* pericardia	The protective sac enclosing the heart composed of two fibrous membranes with fluid between.
	pulmonary semilunar valve	*Syn:* pulmonic valve
40	pulmonic valve; pulmonary valve	The heart valve opening from the right ventricle to the pulmonary artery. See Figure 6. *Syn:* pulmonary semilunar valve
	Purkinje fibers	Specialized cardiac fibers responsible for subendocardial conduction. See Figure 8.
17	right ventricle (RV)	The lower chamber on the right side of the heart that receives the venous blood from the right atrium and drives it into the pulmonary artery by the contraction of its walls. See Figure 6.
26	RV	Abbreviation for right ventricle.
40	semilunar valve	A heart valve composed of a set of three semilunar cusps (valvules); both the aortic and pulmonary valves are semilunar valves. See Figure 6.
17	septum	A wall dividing two cavities or masses of softer tissue. See Figure 6.

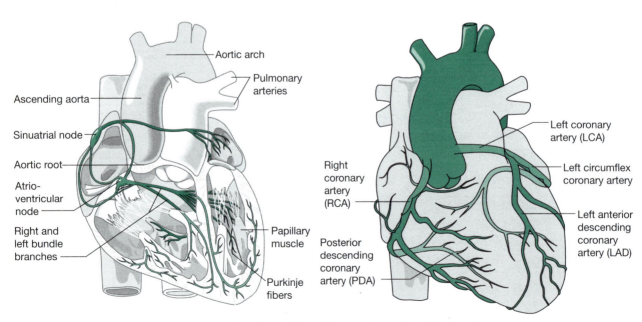

FIGURE 8. The relationship of the great vessels of the heart.

Report #	Term	Definition
17	tricuspid valve	The valve in the orifice between the right atrium and right ventricle of the heart; its three cusps are called anterior, posterior, and septal. See Figure 6.
	trileaflet aortic valve	*Syn:* aortic valve
	valve anulus	The ring portion of the valve.
	valvule	A valve, especially one of small size.
2	ventricle	A normal cavity, as of the heart or brain. In cardiology, the lower chambers of the heart. See Figure 6.
26	ventricular apex	*Syn:* apex
39	ventricular cavity	The hollow space in either of the two lower chambers of the heart. See Figure 6.
	ventricular free walls	The outer walls of the ventricles not associated with the septal regions.
	ventricular outflow tract	The area of the ventricles where blood is channeled out toward the pulmonary or aortic valve.
	ventricular septum	*Syn:* interventricular septum

Vascular anatomy

Report #	Term	Definition
5	abdominal aorta	The part of the descending aorta that supplies structures below the diaphragm.
	anterior interventricular artery	*Syn:* left anterior descending coronary artery
	anterior interventricular branch of the left coronary artery	*Syn:* left anterior descending coronary artery
	anterior jugular vein	Arises below the chin from veins draining the lower lip and mental region, descends the anterior portion of the neck superficial or deep to the investing cervical fascia, and terminates in the external jugular vein at the lateral border of the scalenus anterior muscle.
5	aorta	The main arterial trunk arising from the left ventricle.
18	aortic arch	The curved portion between the ascending and descending parts of the aorta. It gives rise to the brachiocephalic trunk and the left common carotid and left subclavian arteries. See Figure 8.
23	aortic root	The base of the aorta attached to the left ventricle of the heart. See Figure 8.
1	artery, *pl.* arteries	A type of blood vessel transporting oxygenated blood from the heart.

Report #	Term	Definition
27	ascending aorta	The part of the aorta nearest to the aortic arch from which the coronary arteries arise. See Figure 8.
1	carotid artery	See: left common carotid artery, right common carotid artery
	carotid bulb	A slight dilation of the common carotid artery at its bifurcation into external and internal carotids; it contains baroreceptors that, when stimulated, cause slowing of the heart, vasodilation, and a fall in blood pressure.
48	circumflex coronary artery	Terminal branch of the left coronary artery originating in the main left and coursing in the AV groove between the left atrium and the left ventricle, supplying atrial and ventricular branches. See Figure 8. *Syn:* left circumflex artery
8	common carotid artery	See: left common carotid artery, right common carotid artery
5	common femoral artery	*Syn:* femoral artery
30	coronaries	*Syn:* coronary arteries
15	coronary artery, *pl.* coronary arteries	Pertaining to the vessel(s) encircling the heart. See: left coronary artery, right coronary artery
30	coronary ostium	A small opening from the aortic root to the vessels of the heart.
17	descending aorta	A part of the aorta that further divides into the thoracic aorta and continues into the abdominal aorta. See Figure 9.
21	diagonal branch (of an artery)	A directional term used to describe a coronary artery branch; usually a proximal branch of the LAD.
29	dorsalis pedis artery	A continuation of the anterior tibial artery after it crosses the ankle. See Figure 9.
	external jugular vein	A superficial vein formed inferior to the parotid gland by the junction of the posterior auricular vein and the retromandibular vein, and passing down the side of the neck crossing to the sternocleidomastoid muscle vertically to empty into the subclavian vein.
5	femoral artery	A continuation of the external iliac in the upper leg that terminates as the popliteal artery in the knee area. See Figure 9. *Syn:* common femoral artery
	femoral bifurcation	Denoting the branching of the femoral artery.
43	femoral triangle	A triangular space at the upper part of the thigh.
10	femoral vein	A continuation of the popliteal vein as it ascends into the external iliac vein. See Figure 10.
	fibular artery	*Syn:* peroneal artery
10	inferior vena cava	Vein that receives the blood from the lower limbs and the greater part of the pelvic and abdominal organs. See Figure 10.
	innominate veins	Obsolete term for (left and right) brachiocephalic veins.

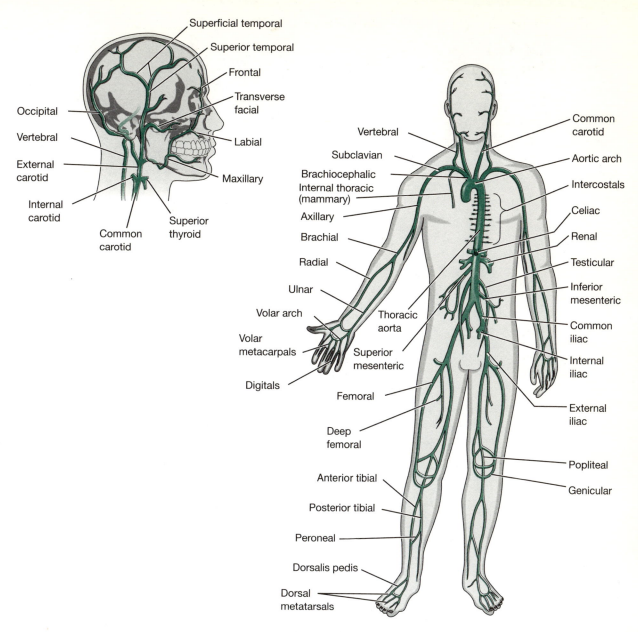

FIGURE 9. Major arteries of the body.

Report #	Term	Definition
1	internal carotid artery	Arises from the common carotid artery opposite the upper border of thyroid cartilage (C-4 vertebral level) and terminates in the middle cranial fossa. See Figure 9.
10	internal jugular vein	Main venous structure of the neck, formed as a continuation of the sigmoid sinus, descending the neck and uniting with the subclavian vein. See Figure 10.
	internal mammary artery	*Syn:* internal thoracic artery

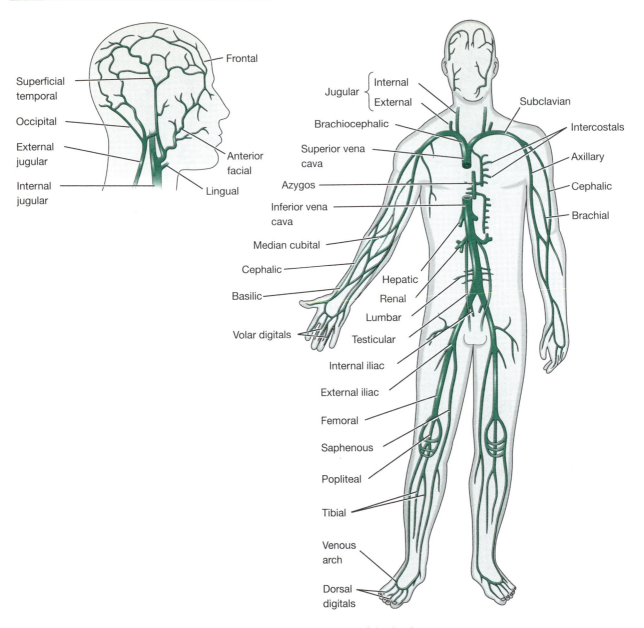

FIGURE 10. Major veins of the body.

Report #	Term	Definition
	internal thoracic artery	Originates from the subclavian artery and descends into the superior epigastric artery. See Figure 9. *Syn:* internal mammary artery
	interventricular septal branches	*Syn:* septal perforating branches
10	jugular vein	See: anterior jugular vein, external jugular vein, internal jugular vein
2	LAD	Abbreviation for left anterior descending (coronary artery).

Report #	Term	Definition
	LCA	Abbreviation for left coronary artery.
2	left anterior descending (LAD) coronary artery	Terminal branch of left coronary artery; originates from left anterior and descends in a groove between the left and right ventricle typically around the apex. See Figure 8. *Syn:* anterior interventricular artery, anterior interventricular branch of left coronary artery
	left circumflex artery	*Syn:* circumflex coronary artery
8	left common carotid artery	The left carotid comes from the arch of the aorta and runs upward, providing blood supply to the neck and head; ascends into internal and external branches. See Figure 9.
2	left coronary artery (LCA)	Originates in the left aortic sinus and divides into two major branches: an anterior ventricular, which descends in the anterior ventricular groove, and a circumflex branch, which passes to the diaphragmatic surface of the left ventricle. See Figure 8.
18	PDA	Abbreviation for posterior descending artery.
	peroneal artery	Originates from the posterior tibial artery and descends to the dorsalis pedis. See Figure 9. *Syn:* fibular artery
29	popliteal artery	A continuation of the femoral artery in the popliteal space, branching off into the anterior and posterior tibial arteries. See Figure 9.
	popliteal vein	Formed by the union of the anterior and posterior tibial veins; ascends through the popliteal space where it continues as the femoral vein. See Figure 10.
43	posterior descending artery (PDA)	Terminal branch of the right coronary artery in posterior interventricular sulcus; descends to the apex. See Figure 8. *Syn:* posterior interventricular branch of the right coronary artery
	posterior interventricular branch of the right coronary artery	*Syn:* posterior descending artery
29	posterior tibial artery	The larger and more directly continuous of the two terminal branches of the popliteal artery. See Figure 9.
23	pulmonary artery	Originates from the right ventricle of the heart and divides into the right pulmonary artery and the left pulmonary artery, which enter the corresponding lungs. See Figure 8.
25	pulmonary veins	Four veins, two on each side, conveying oxygenated blood from the lungs to the left atrium of the heart. *See also:* right superior pulmonary vein. See Figure 6.
30	ramus, *pl.* rami	One of the primary divisions of a nerve or blood vessel.
8	RCA	Abbreviation for right coronary artery.

Report #	Term	Definition
46	right common carotid artery	The right carotid originates from the brachiocephalic trunk and supplies blood to the right side of the head, neck and brain; ascends into internal and external branches. See Figure 9.
2	right coronary artery (RCA)	Originates from the right aortic sinus and passes in the groove between the right atrium and right ventricle, around the right side of the heart, branching to the right atrium and right ventricle. See Figure 8.
27	right superior pulmonary vein	The vein that returns oxygenated blood from the superior and middle lobes of the right lung to the left atrium. See Figure 6.
15	saphenous vein	Formed by the union of the dorsal vein of the great toe and the dorsal venous arch of the foot; ascends into the femoral vein to the upper part of the femoral triangle. See Figure 10.
43	septal perforating branches	Branches of the anterior and posterior descending coronary arteries distributed to the muscle of the interventricular septum. *Syn:* interventricular septal branches
28	subclavian vein	The direct continuation of the axillary vein at the lateral border of the first rib; it passes medially to join the internal jugular vein and forms the brachiocephalic vein on each side. See Figure 10.
42	superficial femoral artery	Portion of the femoral artery situated near the surface.
	superficial femoral vein	Portion of the femoral vein situated near the surface.
	superior epigastric artery	Originates at the medial terminal branch of the internal thoracic artery and supplies blood to the rectus abdominis and the superior part of the anterolateral abdominal wall.
10	superior vena cava	Returns blood from the head and neck, upper limbs and thorax.
	temporal artery	Artery on the side of the head: superficial, middle and deep temporal arteries.
	thoracic aorta	The part of the descending aorta that supplies structures as far down as the diaphragm.
29	tibial artery	Originates from the popliteal forming two branches, posterior and anterior tibial, which both descend to the dorsalis pedis artery. See Figure 9.
10	vein	A type of blood vessel that transports deoxygenated blood from the body tissues to the heart.
1	vertebral artery	The first branch of the subclavian artery which divides into four parts. See Figure 9.

Other related anatomical terms

Report #	Term	Definition
	epigastric area	The region of the abdomen located between the costal margins and the subcostal plane.
	fascia pectoralis	*Syn:* pectoral fascia
	hilum, *pl.* hila	The wedge-shaped depression on the mediastinal surface of each lung, where the bronchus, blood vessels, nerves, and lymphatics enter or leave the lung.
44	medial malleolus	The process at the medial side of the lower end of the tibia, forming the projection of the medial side of the ankle.
27	mediastinal; mediastinum	Pertaining to a septum between two parts of an organ or cavity; the median partition of the thoracic cavity.
4	oropharynx	The portion of the pharynx that lies posterior to the mouth.
30	ostium, *pl.* ostia	A small opening, especially one of entrance into a hollow organ or canal.
28	pectoral fascia	The fascia that covers the pectoralis major muscle. *Syn:* fascia pectoralis
28	prepectoral fascia	The area between the dermis and the pectoral fascia.
	presternal fascia	The fascia over the sternum.
	sternal notch	The large notch in the superior margin of the sternum.
50	subcutaneous tissue	A layer of loose, irregular connective tissue immediately beneath the skin and superficial to the deep fascia, usually consisting primarily of a fatty layer.
49	trapezius muscle	A four-sided muscle of the shoulder with no two sides parallel.
24	xiphoid process	The cartilage at the lower end of the sternum.

Cardiac Symptoms

Report #	Term	Definition
	cardiac syncope	Fainting with loss of consciousness resulting from any cardiac cause. *See also:* syncope
4	chest pain	A general term used to explain multiple sensations in the chest area (e.g., sharp pain, ache, pressure, tightness).
	midsternal chest pain	Pain located at the middle and largest portion of the sternum, lying between the manubrium superiorly and the xiphoid process inferiorly.
16	pleuritic pain	A pain related to inflammation of the pleura.

Report #	Term	Definition
15	radiating	To spread out in all directions from a central point.
	retrosternal chest pain	Pain located posterior to the sternum.
	sharp pain	A pain with sudden onset characterized as stabbing, intense and/or pinching.
	stabbing pain	A pain characterized as brief, repetitive and sharp.
15	substernal chest pain	Pain located below the sternum.
4	syncope; syncopal episode	Fainting and loss of consciousness caused by diminished cerebral blood flow.

Cardiac Conduction and Rhythm Terminology

Report #	Term	Definition
24	amplitude	Relating to the size of the electrocardiogram complex; largeness, extent, breadth or range.
	antitachycardia pacing	A pacing method used to slow down a fast heart rate.
	APC, *pl.* APCs	Abbreviation for atrial premature contraction.
	arrhythmia; arrhythmic	Loss or abnormality of rhythm; denoting especially an irregularity of the heartbeat. *Syn:* dysrhythmia
41	asystole	Absence of contractions of the heart.
	atrial amplitude	The size of the P waves in the electrocardiogram.
11	atrial fibrillation	Rapid irregular atrial twitchings of the atrial myocardium. See Figure 11.
38	atrial flutter	Rapid regular atrial contractions occurring usually at rates between 200 and 330 per minute and often producing "saw-tooth" waves in the electrocardiogram. See Figure 12.
	atrial premature contraction (APC)	*Syn:* premature atrial contraction

FIGURE 11. Atrial fibrillation. Rapid, disorganized atrial activity causes the irregular undulations of the baseline (F waves).

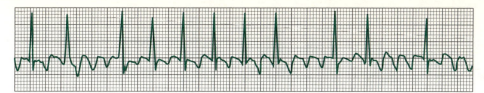

FIGURE 12. Atrial flutter.

Report #	Term	Definition
24	atrioventricular block (AV block)	Partial or complete block of electric impulses originating in the atrium preventing them from reaching the ventricles. See Figure 13.
38	first-degree atrioventricular block	Indicates that there is conduction of the electrical impulses, but a prolonged PR interval.
	second-degree atrioventricular block	Indicates that some but not all atrial impulses fail to reach the ventricles, so some ventricular beats are dropped.
	third-degree atrioventricular block	Complete AV block; no impulses reach the ventricles despite even a slow ventricular rate (under 45 per minute); atria and ventricles beat independently.
33	Wenckebach block	A first-degree atrioventricular block in which there is a progressive lengthening of conduction, as manifested in prolonged P-Q interval on electrocardiography, until one QRS complex and T wave are missed.
	AV block	Abbreviation for atrioventricular block.
	AV delay	A marked delay in the electric impulse traveling from the sinus node to the AV node and ventricles.
18	axis deviation	Deflection of the electrical axis of the heart to the right or left of the normal.
	left axis deviation	A mean electrical axis of the heart pointing to -30° or more negative.
	right axis deviation	A mean electrical axis of the heart pointing to the right of +90°.
	bigeminal rhythm	Paired ventricular beats, consisting of ventricular extrasystoles coupled to sinus beats. See Figure 14.
	blanking period	The period of time after the paced beat when the pacemaker will ignore any signal; lasts from 200 to 300 msec.

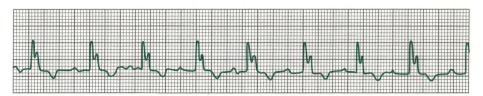

FIGURE 13. Heart block.

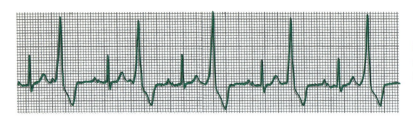

FIGURE 14. Ventricular bigeminy. QRS complexes alternate between sinus beats and ventricular premature systoles.

Report #	Term	Definition
19	bradycardia	Slowness of the heartbeat, usually defined (by convention) as a rate under 50 beats per minute. See Figure 15.
38	bundle-branch block	Intraventricular block due to interruption of conduction in one of the two main branches (left or right) of the bundle of His and manifested in the electrocardiogram by marked prolongation of the QRS complex.
28	capture; capturing	Conduction of a pacemaker-generated impulse through the myocardium as represented on an electrocardiogram.
	cardiac arrest	Complete cessation of cardiac activity either electric, mechanical or both; may be purposely induced for therapeutic reasons.
	cardiac sounds	*Syn:* heart sounds
24	complex	An electrocardiogram waveform representing the electrical activity of the heart.
28	defibrillation	The electrical termination of fibrillation of the cardiac muscle.
	dysrhythmia	*Syn:* arrhythmia
7	ectopic	Denoting a heartbeat that has its origin in some focus other than the sinuatrial node.
	extrasystole	A premature heartbeat.
	frontal axis	A description of the heart's assumed electrical characteristics based on the form of the QRS complexes in limb leads.
2	heart block	*Syn:* atrioventricular block
16	heart sounds	The noise made by muscle contraction and the closure of the heart valves during the cardiac cycle. See Figure 16. *Syn:* cardiac sounds, heart tones
	first heart sound (S_1)	Occurs with ventricular systole and is mainly produced by closure of the atrioventricular valves.

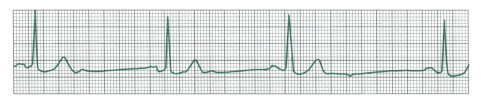

FIGURE 15. Bradycardia.

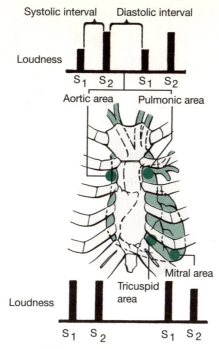

FIGURE 16. Heart sounds.

Report #	Term	Definition
16	second heart sound (S₂)	Signifies the beginning of diastole and is due to closure of the semilunar valves.
	third heart sound (S₃)	Occurs in early diastole and corresponds with the end of the first phase of rapid ventricular filling; normal in children and younger people but abnormal in others.
	fourth heart sound (S₄)	Produced in late diastole in association with ventricular filling due to atrial systole and related to reduced ventricular compliance. It is common in ventricular hypertrophy, particularly with hypertension. *Syn:* atrial sound
	atrial sound	*Syn:* fourth heart sound (S₄)
	prosthetic S₂	The second heart sound made by the prosthetic heart valve.
	heart tones	*Syn:* heart sounds
24	impedance	A measurement of the electrical energy needed to stimulate myocardial tissue.
7	interval	The time elapsing between two consecutive electrocardiogram complexes in the electrocardiogram.
26	AH interval, A-H interval	The time from the initial rapid deflection of the atrial wave to the initial rapid deflection of the His bundle (H) potential.
	AV interval, A-V interval	The time from the beginning of atrial systole to the beginning of ventricular systole as measured from pressure pulses or cardiac volume curves in animals, or from the electrocardiogram in humans.

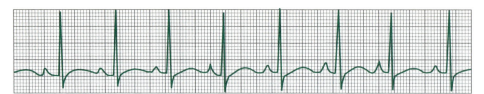

FIGURE 17. Normal sinus rhythm (NSR).

Report #	Term	Definition
26	HV interval, H-V interval	The time from the initial deflection of the His bundle (H) potential and the onset of ventricular activity.
7	PR interval, P-R interval	The time elapsing between the beginning of the P wave and the beginning of the next QRS complex.
28	joule	A unit of energy; the heat generated, or energy expended, by an ampere flowing through an ohm for 1 second.
4	normal sinus rhythm (NSR)	Cardiac rhythm proceeding from the sinuatrial node; in healthy adults its rate is 60 to 90 beats per minute. See Figure 17. *Syn:* sinus rhythm
	NSR	Abbreviation for normal sinus rhythm.
	P-wave amplitude	The vertical size of the first complex of the electrocardiogram, during sinus and atrial rhythms, representing depolarization of the atria. See Figure 18.

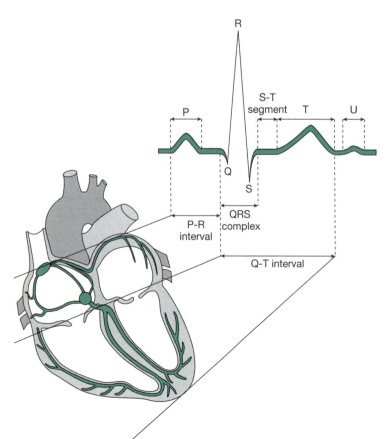

FIGURE 18. An electrical picture of the heart is represented by positive and negative deflections on a graph labeled with the letters P, Q, R, S and T, corresponding to the events of the cardiac cycle.

Report #	Term	Definition
8	PAC, *pl.* PACs	Abbreviation for premature atrial contraction.
	pacing mode	A programmed set of instructions in a pacemaker generator on how and when to send an impulse to the heart.
	DDD pacing mode	A pacing mode with *d*ual (i.e., atrial and ventricular) chamber pacing, *d*ual chamber sensing and *d*ual chamber response to sensing that either triggers or inhibits pacing.
	DDDR pacing mode	Identical to the DDD pacing mode with the added feature of *rate* response.
	VVIR pacing mode	A pacing mode in which the *v*entricle is paced, the *v*entricle is sensing, there is an *i*nhibited response to sensing and it is *r*ate responsive.
24	pacing threshold	The minimal pacemaker-generated stimulus that produces excitation of the myocardium.
4	palpitation	Forcible or irregular pulsation of the heart, perceptible to the patient, usually with an increase in frequency or force, with or without irregularity in rhythm.
	parameters	A way of measuring or describing electrocardiographic complexes.
19	pause	A temporary delay or slowing between heart contractions.
	premature atrial contraction (PAC)	An early contraction of the atria, represented by a P wave close to or during the repolarization phase. See Figure 19. *Syn:* atrial premature contraction
	premature ventricular contraction (PVC)	An early contraction of the ventricles, represented by a QRS wave close to or during the repolarization phase. See Figure 20. *Syn:* ventricular premature contraction
	pulse wave	The progressive expansion of the arteries occurring with each contraction of the left ventricle of the heart.
	pulse wave duration	*Syn:* pulse width
28	pulse width	The interval between onset of the leading edge and the end of the trailing edge of the electrocardiogram complex. *Syn:* pulse wave duration

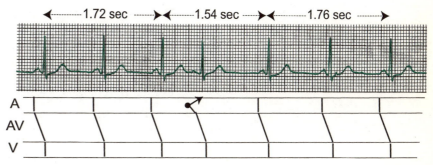

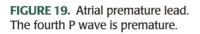

FIGURE 19. Atrial premature lead. The fourth P wave is premature.

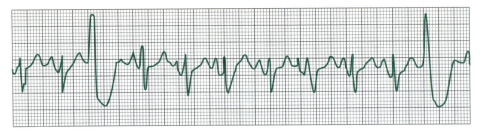

FIGURE 20. Premature ventricular contraction (PVC).

Report #	Term	Definition
	PVC, *pl.* PVCs	Abbreviation for premature ventricular contraction.
30	QRS complex	The portion of the electrocardiogram corresponding to the depolarization of ventricular cardiac cells.
	rate response	A feature of a pacemaker generator that monitors the intrinsic heart rate needs and adjusts the rate accordingly.
37	resistance	A measurement of force exerted in opposition to an active force.
	retrograde conduction	A heartbeat occurring in the reverse order (e.g., an atrial beat triggered by an impulse originating in the ventricle).
	right-to-left shunt	The passage of blood from the right side of the heart into the left (as through a septal defect), or from the pulmonary artery into the aorta (as through a patent ductus arteriosus); such a shunt can occur only when the pressure on the right side exceeds that in the left.
	segment	In electrocardiography, a specific portion of an electrocardiogram tracing.
2	ST segment	The part of the electrocardiogram between the QRS complex and the T wave; represents completion of depolarization and the beginning of repolarization. See Figure 18.
37	sensitivity	The ability to respond to a stimulus.
50	shock on T-wave algorithm	An electrical impulse delivered to the heart while in the refractory period (T wave), which can cause a ventricular fibrillation or tachycardic arrhythmia.
7	sinus rhythm	*Syn:* normal sinus rhythm
26	stimulation	The application of a stimulus to a responsive structure, such as the myocardium, regardless of whether the strength of the stimulus is sufficient to produce excitation.
7	tachycardia	Rapid beating of the heart, conventionally applied to rates exceeding 100 beats per minute.
50	monomorphic ventricular tachycardia	A heart rate between 120 and 240 beats per minute with identical wide QRS morphology.

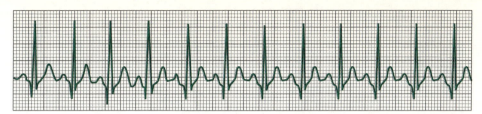

FIGURE 21. Sinus tachycardia.

Report #	Term	Definition
	paroxysmal supraventricular tachycardia (PST, PSVT)	Recurrent attacks of tachycardia, usually with abrupt onset and often also with abrupt termination, originating from an ectopic focus that may be atrial, AV junctional or ventricular.
16	PST; PSVT	Abbreviations for paroxysmal supraventricular tachycardia.
	sinus tachycardia	A fast heart rate originating in the sinus node. See Figure 21.
33	supraventricular tachycardia (SVT)	Rapid heart rate (greater than 100 beats per minute) anywhere above the ventricular level (i.e., sinus node, atrium, atrioventricular junction).
33	SVT, *pl.* SVTs	Abbreviation for supraventricular tachycardia.
7	ventricular tachycardia (VT)	Rapid rhythm originating in the ventricles (either the bundle branches of the Purkinje system or ventricular muscle).
10	VT	Abbreviation for ventricular tachycardia.
	wide-complex tachycardia	A fast heart rate in which the QRS complexes are not narrow (greater than 120 msec) suggesting that there is either supraventricular origin with rate-related aberrancy or preexisting intraventricular conduction delay of ventricular origin. See Figure 22.
	tachycardic	Relating to rapid heart rate.
24	threshold	The point at which a stimulus first produces a response.
	trigeminal rhythm	A cardiac arrhythmia in which the beats are grouped in trios, usually composed of a sinus beat followed by two extrasystoles.
50	ventricular capture	Response of the ventricle(s) by an impulse arising in the atria or AV junction.
2	ventricular fibrillation (VF)	Coarse or fine, rapid, fibrillary movements of the ventricular muscle that replace the normal contraction. See Figure 23.

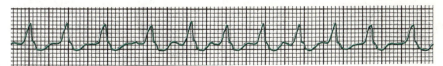

FIGURE 22. Wide-complex tachycardia.

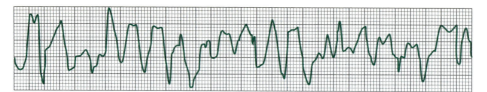

FIGURE 23. Ventricular fibrillation.

Report #	Term	Definition
	ventricular premature contraction	*Syn:* premature ventricular contraction
	VF	Abbreviation for ventricular fibrillation.
50	volt resistance	A measurement of the electrical force exerted in opposition to an active force.
28	voltage	Electromotive force, pressure or potential expressed in volts.
	VPC, *pl.* VPCs	Abbreviation for ventricular premature contraction.
	wave	In electrocardiography, a deflection of special shape and extent in the electrocardiogram representing the electric activity of a portion of the heart muscle.
	A wave	An atrial deflection in an electrogram recorded from within the atrium of the heart; the first positive deflection of the atrial and venous pulses due to atrial systole.
28, 38	P wave	The portion of the electrocardiogram representing atrial depolarization.
	Q wave	The initial deflection of the QRS complex when such deflection is negative (downward). See Figure 18.
	QRS wave	The portion of the electrocardiogram corresponding to the ventricular depolarization associated with ventricular contraction. See Figure 18.
24	R wave	The first positive (upward) deflection of the QRS complex in the electrocardiogram, corresponding to ventricular depolarization. See Figure 18.
13	T wave	Waveform in an electrocardiogram tracing representing ventricular repolarization. See Figure 18.
	U wave	Waveform in an electrocardiogram following the T wave that represents repolarization of the ventricular Purkinje fibers. See Figure 18.
	V wave	A large pressure wave visible in recordings from either atrium or its incoming veins, normally produced by venous return.
26, 41	Wenckebach cycle	A sequence of cardiac cycles in the electrocardiogram ending in a dropped beat due to AV block, the preceding cycles showing progressively lengthening PR intervals; the PR interval following the dropped beat is again shortened.

Diagnoses

Report #	Term	Definition
	AAA	Abbreviation for abdominal aortic aneurysm; commonly dictated "triple A."
15	abdominal aortic aneurysm (AAA)	Circumscribed dilation of the abdominal aorta usually due to an acquired or congenital weakness of the wall of the vessel.
	ACS	Abbreviation for acute coronary syndrome.
	acute anterior myocardial infarction	A heart attack of rapid onset due to the lack of oxygenated blood to the front and interior cardiac wall.
	acute coronary syndrome (ACS)	Rapid onset of chest pain associated with decreased blood flow to the heart.
	acute endocardial myocardial infarction	A heart attack due to a lack of blood supply to the innermost tunic of the heart.
4	anemia	Any condition in which there is a reduction in the number of red blood cells, the amount of hemoglobin and/or the volume of packed red blood cells, resulting in a lack of oxygen being transported to body tissues.
2	aneurysm	Circumscribed dilation of an artery or a cardiac chamber, usually due to an acquired or congenital weakness of the wall of the artery or chamber. See Figure 24.
	aneurysmal redundant segment	Repeated sections of arterial wall dilations.
2	angina; angina pectoris	Severe constricting pain in the chest, often radiating from the precordium to a shoulder (usually left) and down the arm, due to ischemia of the heart muscle usually caused by coronary disease.

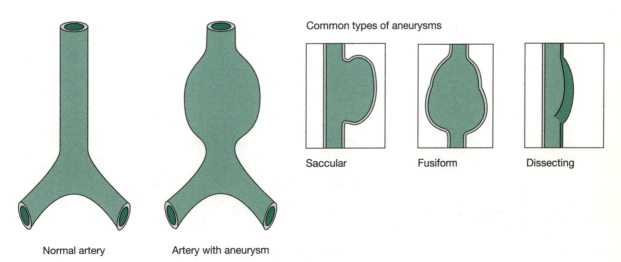

Common types of aneurysms

Saccular   Fusiform   Dissecting

Normal artery   Artery with aneurysm

FIGURE 24. Types of aneurysms.

Report #	Term	Definition
34	aortic insufficiency	Reflux of blood through an incompetent aortic valve into the left ventricle during ventricular diastole.
40	aortic root sclerosis	Hardening of the aortic vessel wall connecting to the left ventricle.
	arteriosclerotic cardiovascular disease (ASCVD)	The most common type of aneurysm, occurring in the abdominal aorta and other large arteries, primarily in the elderly.
	ASCVD	Abbreviation for arteriosclerotic cardiovascular disease.
34	ASD	Abbreviation for atrial septal defect.
44	atherosclerosis	A build-up of plaque that in time becomes fibrous and may calcify, causing narrowing and hardening of the vessel walls.
30	atrial septal defect (ASD)	An opening in the septum separating the atria.
	CAD	Abbreviation for coronary artery disease.
	cardiomegaly	Enlargement of the heart.
2	cardiomyopathy	Disease of the myocardium.
	cardioneurogenic syncope	Fainting with unconsciousness resulting from any cardiac or neural cause.
	cardiopulmonary arrest	The absence of cardiac and pulmonary activity.
15	carotid bruit	A systolic murmur heard in the neck but not at the aortic area; any bruit produced by turbulent blood flow in a carotid artery.
	cerebrovascular accident (CVA)	An imprecise term for cerebral stroke; any acute clinical event related to impairment of cerebral circulation that lasts more than 24 hours.
13	CHF	Abbreviation for congestive heart failure.
	common iliac artery aneurysm	A dilation or weakening of the artery branching off the terminal end of the abdominal aorta.
9	congestive heart failure (CHF)	Inadequacy of the pumping action of the heart, failing to maintain the circulation of blood, resulting in congestion and edema of the tissues. *Syn:* heart failure
8	coronary artery disease (CAD)	A pathologic state causing decreased blood flow to the myocardium.
8	CVA	Abbreviation for cerebrovascular accident.
13	deep vein thrombosis	The development of blood clots in the deep veins of the legs, pelvis or arms.
	diaphragmatic myocardial infarction	*Syn:* inferior myocardial infarction
6	diastolic dysfunction	Abnormal postsystolic dilation of the heart cavities, during which they fill with blood.

Report #	Term	Definition
	diffuse left ventricular dysfunction	Inability of the left heart to maintain efficient circulation.
40	dilated cardiomyopathy	Diseased enlargement of the heart muscle.
	dilated foramen ovale	An enlarged opening between the right and left atria which usually closes during the birth process when the newborn takes its first breath.
48	fascicular block	A condition due to conduction delay in one of the two major fascicles of the left bundle branch.
40	fibrocalcific changes of the aortic and mitral valve	A build-up of plaque that becomes fibrous and calcifies, causing narrowing and hardening of the affected valves.
	heart attack	*Syn:* myocardial infarction
9	heart failure	*Syn:* congestive heart failure
	hypercalcemia	The presence of an abnormally large amount of calcium in the blood.
	hypercholesterolemia	The presence of an abnormally large amount of cholesterol in the blood.
	hyperglycemia	The presence of an abnormally large amount of glucose in the blood.
	hyperkalemia	The presence of an abnormally large amount of potassium in the blood.
9	hyperlipidemia	The presence of an abnormally high concentration of lipids in the circulating blood. *Syn:* lipemia
	hypernatremia	The presence of an abnormally large amount of sodium in the blood.
4	hypertension	High blood pressure.
	hypoglycemia	A deficiency of glucose in the blood.
	impaired ventricular systolic function	Pathologic interference in the contraction of the ventricles. *Syn:* ventricular systolic dysfunction
	inducible myocardial ischemia	A lack of blood flow to the heart usually as a result of occlusion of a coronary artery.
2	infarction	An insufficiency of arterial blood supply due to emboli, thrombi, mechanical factors or pressure that produces necrosis; any organ can be affected. See Figure 25.
15	inferior myocardial infarction	Infarction involving the inferior or diaphragmatic wall of the heart, producing indicative changes in leads II, III, and aVF in the electrocardiogram. *Syn:* diaphragmatic myocardial infarction
6	intracardiac mass	A lump or aggregation of adherent material located within the heart.

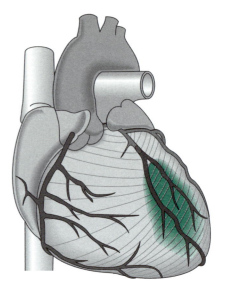

FIGURE 25. Anterolateral myocardial infarction (darkened area), caused by occlusion of the anterior descending branch of the left coronary artery.

Report #	Term	Definition
	intracardiac thrombus	A blood clot within the heart.
2, 21	ischemia; ischemic	A decrease in blood supply to tissue due to vessel obstruction or blockage.
26	ischemic cardiomyopathy	Disease of the myocardium caused by a lack of blood supply to the area.
4	jugular venous distention (JVD)	A condition characterized by the stretching or prominence of the jugular vein.
4	JVD	Abbreviation for jugular venous distention.
6	left ventricular hypertrophy (LVH)	Abnormal enlargement of the left ventricle.
	lipemia	*Syn:* hyperlipidemia
	LVH	Abbreviation for left ventricular hypertrophy.
	LVH with flattening	Description of the left ventricular wall motion on echographic study.
17	mitral regurgitation	Reflux of blood through an incompetent mitral valve.
2	myocardial infarction	Insufficiency of coronary artery blood supply to the heart muscle resulting in tissue death. *Syn:* heart attack
	near-syncopal episode	Episode where patient feels as if he or she will faint, but without loss of consciousness.
	neurogenic syncope	Fainting with a neurologic cause.
	paradoxical embolus	Obstruction of an artery by an embolus from a vein that passes through a septal defect, patent foramen ovale or other shunt to the arterial system.
6	pericardial effusion	Increased fluid within the pericardial sac.
16	pericarditis	Inflammation of the membrane surrounding the heart.

Report #	Term	Definition
13	peripheral vascular disease (PVD)	An abnormal condition affecting blood vessels other than the heart.
	pharmacologic stress-induced ischemia	Lack of blood flow caused by drugs that put pressure on the cardiovascular system.
	phlebitis	Inflammation of a vein.
	posterior myocardial infarction	Infarction involving the posterior wall of the heart.
	postural hypotension	A form of low blood pressure that occurs with a patient in a standing posture.
	primary arrhythmic event	A main irregular heart rhythm.
	PVD	Abbreviation for peripheral vascular disease.
4	rhonchus, *pl.* rhonchi	An added sound with a musical pitch occurring during inspiration or expiration, heard on auscultation of the chest, and caused by air passing through bronchi that are narrowed by inflammation, spasm of smooth muscle or presence of mucus in the lumen; if low-pitched, it is called sonorous rhonchus; if high-pitched with a whistling or squeaky quality, sibilant rhonchus.
38	right bundle-branch block	Intraventricular block of the conduction impulse due to interruption in the right branch of the two main branches of the His bundle.
	sick sinus syndrome (SSS)	Symptoms ranging from dizziness to unconsciousness due to chaotic or absent atrial activity often with bradycardia alternating with tachycardia, recurring ectopic beats including escape beats, runs of supraventricular and ventricular arrhythmias, sinus arrest and sinuatrial block.
	sinus tachycardia with left bundle-branch block	Tachycardia originating in the sinus node with a delay of the impulse going through the left branch of the bundle of His.
	SSS	Abbreviation for sick sinus syndrome.
	stress ischemia	Lack of blood flow caused by stress or pressure on the cardiovascular system.
	symptomatic bradycardia	Slow heart rate with symptoms.
	temporal arteritis	Vessel inflammation or infection involving the temporal artery.
13	thrombosis	The development of blood clots.
17	tricuspid regurgitation	The backward flow through the valve closing the orifice between the right atrium and right ventricle of the heart.
40	valvular vegetation	A clot, composed largely of fused blood platelets, fibrin and sometimes microorganisms, adherent to a diseased heart valve and often initiated by infection of the structures involved.

Report #	Term	Definition
	ventricular rupture	A tear in the wall of the ventricle.
48	ventricular systolic dysfunction	*Syn:* impaired ventricular systolic function

Diagnostic Procedures

Invasive, surgical terms

Report #	Term	Definition
29	angiogram	A radiograph obtained by angiography.
2	angiography	Radiography of vessels after injection of a radiopaque contrast material; usually involves percutaneous insertion of a radiopaque catheter and positioning under fluoroscopic control.
	arteriogram	Radiographic demonstration of an artery after injection of contrast medium.
8	arteriography	Visualization of an artery or arteries by x-ray imaging after injection of a radiopaque contrast medium.
	biopsy	Process of removing tissue for diagnostic examination.
2	cardiac catheterization	Procedure in which a thin plastic tube is inserted into an artery or vein in the arm or leg and advanced to the chambers of the heart or the coronary arteries.
48	conscious sedation	A medically controlled state of depressed consciousness in which airway patency, protective reflexes and the ability to respond to stimulation or verbal commands are preserved.
43	coronary angiography	Imaging of the circulation of the myocardium by injection of contrast medium, usually by selective catheterization of each coronary artery, formerly by nonselective injection at the root of the aorta.
48	coronary arteriography	Visualization of the coronary arteries by x-ray imaging after injection of a radiopaque contrast medium.
	digital subtraction angiography (DSA)	Computer-assisted radiographic angiography permitting visualization of vascular structures without superimposed bone and soft tissue densities.
	DSA	Abbreviation for digital subtraction angiography.
26	electrophysiologic study (EP)	Procedure where catheters are inserted into the right or left atrium and used to pace the heart and potentially induce arrhythmias to identify defects in the heart. Also used therapeutically to stop arrhythmias.
	EP	Abbreviation for electrophysiologic study.

Report #	Term	Definition
	femoral angiography	Radiography of the femoral vessels after the injection of a radiopaque contrast material. *Syn:* femoral arteriography
	femoral arteriography	*Syn:* femoral angiography
43	Judkins technique	A method of selective coronary artery catheterization utilizing the standard Seldinger technique through a percutaneous femoral artery puncture. *Syn:* standard Judkins technique
21	left heart catheterization	Radiography of the left ventricle and coronary arteries after the injection of a radiopaque contrast material to determine plaque, strictures or other arterial blockages. In comparison, right heart catheterization is used to measure pressure within the arteries.
43	left internal mammary graft angiography	Radiography of the left internal mammary artery after the injection of a radiopaque contrast material.
	modified Seldinger technique	A method with some changes to percutaneous insertion of a catheter into a blood vessel or space. A needle is used to puncture the structure and a guidewire is threaded through the needle. When the needle is withdrawn, a catheter is threaded over the wire. The wire is then withdrawn, leaving the catheter in place. *See also:* Seldinger technique
	post-stent angiography	Radiography of an artery with a stent after the injection of a radiopaque contrast material.
	right heart catheterization	Catheterization of the right heart to measure pressures, output, index/indices and saturations, and as a means to determine if a patient has pulmonary hypertension; usually done on patients with CHF, COPD or other chronic pulmonary diseases. In comparison, left heart catheterization is performed to determine arterial blockages or strictures.
43	saphenous vein graft angiography	Radiography of a saphenous vein bypass graft after the injection of a radiopaque contrast material.
5	Seldinger technique	A method of percutaneous insertion of a catheter into a blood vessel or space. A needle is used to puncture the structure and a guidewire is threaded through the needle. When the needle is withdrawn, a catheter is threaded over the wire. The wire is then withdrawn, leaving the catheter in place. *See also:* modified Seldinger technique
43	standard Judkins technique	*Syn:* Judkins technique
	temporal artery biopsy	Process of removing tissue from a temporal artery for diagnostic examination.
2	ventriculography (right and left)	Demonstration of the contractility of the cardiac ventricles by serially recording the distribution of an intravenously injected radionuclide or that of radiographic contrast medium injected through an intracardiac catheter.

Noninvasive terms

Report #	Term	Definition
14	Bruce protocol	A standardized protocol for electrocardiogram-monitored exercise using increasing speeds and elevations of the treadmill. *Syn:* standard Bruce protocol
11	ECG	The more commonly used abbreviation for electrocardiogram.
12	EKG	The less commonly used abbreviation for electrocardiogram.
	electrocardiogram (ECG, EKG)	An electrical picture of the heart represented by positive and negative deflections on a graph labeled with the letters P, Q, R, S and T, each of which corresponds to events of the cardiac cycle. See Figure 18.
	electrocardiography	The process of recording the electrical conductivity of the heart.
25	fluoroscopy	Examination of the tissues and deep structures of the body by x-ray, using the fluoroscope or video fluoroscopy.
7	Holter monitor	A technique for long-term and continuous, usually ambulatory, recording of electrocardiographic signals on magnetic tape.
	12-lead electrocardiograph	Recordings via electrodes placed at particular points on the body surface to produce 12 perspectives of the cardiac electrical activity.
	resting ECG, resting EKG	An electrocardiogram performed when the patient is at rest.
14	standard Bruce protocol	*Syn:* Bruce protocol
	stress electrocardiogram	An electrocardiogram performed when the patient is exercising on a treadmill or when the patient's heart is being stimulated pharmacologically.
19	tilt table test	A test that involves monitoring the cardiac response when the body is inverted, head down; used to study the response of the circulatory system to gravitational force.

Radiology terms

Report #	Term	Definition
11	chest x-ray	A radiographic picture of the organs and structures within the chest cavity.
	cut film	In radiology, refers to an x-ray on a piece of film.
6	Doppler study	A diagnostic method that involves passing an ultrasonic beam into the body; Doppler-created ultrasound makes possible real-time viewing of tissues, blood flow and organs that cannot be observed by any other method.
39	color Doppler flow	A computer-generated color image produced by Doppler ultrasonography in which different directions of flow are represented in different hues.

Report #	Term	Definition
	color venous duplex	A method of visualizing and selectively assessing the flow patterns of peripheral veins using ultrasound imaging and pulsed color Doppler.
6	Doppler echocardiography	Use of Doppler ultrasonography techniques to augment two-dimensional echocardiography by allowing velocities to be registered within the echocardiographic image.
	duplex Doppler scan	A method of visualizing and selectively assessing the flow patterns of peripheral arteries and veins using ultrasound imaging and pulsed Doppler.
6	echocardiography	The use of ultrasound in the investigation of the heart and great vessels and diagnosis of cardiovascular lesions.
	contrast bubble study	*Syn:* contrast echocardiography
	contrast echocardiography	An injection of saline with tiny bubbles used during an echocardiogram to determine whether an abnormal opening is present between the right and left sides of the heart. *Syn:* contrast bubble study
	cross-sectional echocardiography	*Syn:* two-dimensional echocardiography
6, 23, 39	M-mode echocardiography	A single dimension ultrasound of the heart for accurate measurement of the chambers.
	real-time echocardiography	*Syn:* two-dimensional echocardiography
17	TEE	Abbreviation for transesophageal echocardiography.
17	transesophageal echocardiography (TEE)	Recording of the echocardiogram from a transducer swallowed by the patient to predetermined distances in the esophagus and stomach.
6, 22, 23, 39	two-dimensional echocardiography	A two-dimensional videotape ultrasound that displays a cross-sectional view of the beating heart. *Syn:* cross-sectional echocardiography, real-time echocardiography
	thrombolysis in myocardial infarction (TIMI)	An index or measurement of blood flow in acute coronary syndromes, in which a grade number designates the level of perfusion: grade 0 = no flow; grade 1 = penetration without perfusion; grade 2 = partial perfusion; grade 3 = complete perfusion.
	TIMI	Abbreviation for thrombolysis in myocardial infarction.

Common nuclear medicine terms

Report #	Term	Definition
	Cardiolite treadmill	A nuclear perfusion study in conjunction with stress testing to assess the coronary arteries after injection of the radioactive substance Cardiolite (technetium-99m sestamibi).

Report #	Term	Definition
48	filling defect	Displacement of contrast medium by a space-occupying lesion in a radiographic study of a contrast-filled hollow viscus, such as a polyp on a barium enema; also applied to defects in the otherwise uniform distribution of radionuclide in an organ, such as a metastasis in the liver on a ^{99m}Tc-sulfur colloid scan.
	MIBI stress test	Another name used for a technetium-99m sestamibi scan or thallium scan.
	multiple-gated acquisition scan (MUGA scan)	A nuclear study involving the injection of technetium-99m for ejection fraction and wall motion assessment.
	myocardial perfusion study	A type of nuclear study done with radioactive substances to assess heart function.
14	nuclear imaging	A general term for imaging studies done with radioactive substances.
15	nuclear stress test	A study that incorporates both stress testing and radioactive substances to assess heart function.
	pharmacological study	Any study in which the heart is stressed by pharmacologic means rather than exercise.
	single photon emission computed tomography (SPECT)	Positron emission tomography (PET) imaging after the administration of a radionuclide; used to screen for coronary artery disease, to assess flow rates and flow reserve, and to distinguish viable from nonviable myocardium in bypass and transplant candidates.
	SPECT	Abbreviation for single photon emission computed tomography.
	technetium-99m (^{99m}Tc, Tc-99m)	A radioisotope of technetium that decays by isomeric transition, and is used to prepare radiopharmaceuticals for scanning the brain, parotid, thyroid, lungs, blood pool, liver, heart, spleen, kidney, lacrimal drainage apparatus, bone and bone marrow.
	^{99m}Tc sestamibi	A radioactive material of technetium used in nuclear perfusion studies to assess coronary artery occlusion. Cardiolite is a brand name version of this material.
	^{99m}Tc pyrophosphate	A radionuclide tracer used for imaging ischemic myocardium in nuclear medicine.
12, 14	thallium stress echocardiogram	A nuclear perfusion study in conjunction with stress testing and echocardiography to assess the coronary arteries after injection of the radioactive substance.

Laboratory values related to cardiovascular medicine

Report #	Term	Definition	Normal Range of Results
	ABG	Abbreviation for arterial blood gas.	
	ACT	Abbreviation for activated clotting time.	

Report #	Term	Definition	Normal Range of Results
	activated clotting time (ACT)	The most common test used for coagulation time in cardiovascular surgery.	monitored by physician during procedure
	arterial blood gas (ABG) analysis	A clinical expression for partial pressures of oxygen (O) and carbon dioxide (CO_2) in the arterial blood; used to gather information regarding the acid-base status of the patient. *Syn:* blood gas	CO_2: 36–46 mmHg O: 74–109 mmHg
	bicarbonate	A central buffering agent in the blood; values are typically tested as part of an electrolyte panel to check for an electrolyte or pH imbalance.	24–31 mEq/L
	blood gas	*Syn:* arterial blood gas analysis	
	blood urea nitrogen (BUN)	Nitrogen, in the form of urea, in the blood; the most prevalent of nonprotein nitrogenous compounds in blood; values are commonly used as a measure of renal function.	8–18 mg/dL
4	BUN	Abbreviation for blood urea nitrogen.	
	Ca	Abbreviation for calcium.	
	calcium (Ca)	An electrolyte that functions in blood clotting, nerve conduction and muscle contraction; it is also important in bone and teeth formation.	8.8–10.3 mg/dL
	carbon dioxide content	A blood test used to assess carbon dioxide level in the blood.	24–31 mEq/L
	cardiac enzyme study	A measurement of the levels of troponin, creatine phosphokinase and lactate dehydrogenase in the blood. High levels may signal cardiac muscle or other tissue damage.	various references
9	CBC	Abbreviation for complete blood count.	
	chemistry profile	A set of tests to evaluate the body's electrolyte balance and the status of several major body organs; used to assess overall health and well-being.	various references
4	chloride (Cl)	An electrolyte that functions to maintain balance of body fluids and hydrochloric acid in the stomach.	97–107 mEq/L
	Cl	Abbreviation for chloride.	
	CK	Abbreviation for creatine phosphokinase.	
	CK-MB	An isoenzyme of creatine kinase found in cardiac muscle, tongue, diaphragm and in small amounts in skeletal muscle; values serve as an important marker following myocardial infarctions. *See also:* MB index	0–7 ng/mL

Report #	Term	Definition	Normal Range of Results
	CO_2	The chemical formula for carbon dioxide.	
	complete blood count (CBC)	A count of the cells in the blood, including red blood cell indices and count, white blood cell count, hematocrit, hemoglobin, platelets and differential blood count, conveying information on the number, type, size, shape and other physical characteristics of the cells.	various references
	comprehensive metabolic panel	A group of 14 specific tests that provide information about the kidneys, liver, electrolytes, pH balance, blood sugar and blood protein.	various references
	CPK	Abbreviation for creatine phosphokinase.	
	creatine kinase (CK)	A cardiac enzyme; high levels in the blood may reflect heart muscle damage.	females: 30–135 IU/L males: 55–170 IU/L
	creatine phosphokinase (CPK)	Obsolete name for creatine kinase.	
4	creatinine	Usually reviewed in conjunction with blood urea nitrogen to assess kidney function.	females: 0.6–1.1 mg/dL males: 0.7–1.3 mg/dL
15	digoxin	A cardioactive steroid glycoside obtained from the *Digitalis lanata* plant. Administered as a drug to treat congestive heart failure; serum digoxin levels must be monitored to avoid drug toxicity.	0.5–2.0 ng/mL
	erythrocyte	A mature red blood cell that transports oxygen bound to hemoglobin throughout the circulatory system; erythrocyte indices determine the average size, hemoglobin content and concentration of hemoglobin in red blood cells.	*see* red blood cell count
	lipid profile	A set of tests to evaluate coronary heart disease risk; typically includes high-density lipoprotein cholesterol, low-density lipoprotein cholesterol, total cholesterol and triglyceride levels.	various references
4	glucose; blood glucose	A simple sugar that circulates in the blood as a nutrient for cells; abnormal results indicate a problem with glucose metabolism.	65–110 mg/dL
	HCT	Abbreviation for hematocrit.	
4	hematocrit (HCT)	Percentage of the volume of a blood sample occupied by cells; used to assess the extent of blood loss and of normal hydration levels.	females: 37–47% males: 42–52% children: 30–53% newborns: 53–65%

Report #	Term	Definition	Normal Range of Results
4	hemoglobin (HGB)	The red respiratory protein of red blood cells that transports oxygen from the lungs to the tissues where the oxygen is readily released.	females: 12–16 g/dL males: 14–18 g/dL children: 11.2–16.5 g/dL newborns: 17–23 g/dL
	HGB	Abbreviation for hemoglobin.	
13	INR	Abbreviation for international normalized ratio.	
13	international normalized ratio (INR)	The prothrombin time ratio that would have been obtained if a standard reagent had been used in a prothrombin time determination.	2–3 seconds for patients on Coumadin therapy 2.5–3.5 for patients with prosthetic heart valves
	K	Abbreviation for potassium.	
	LET	Abbreviation for leukocyte esterase test.	
	leukocyte	A white blood cell; protects against pathogens and can be found in blood, tissues and the lymphatic system.	*see* white blood cell count
	leukocyte esterase test (LET)	A chemical assay to determine the presence of lysed or intact white blood cells in urine; used to screen for asymptomatic urinary tract infections.	positive/negative
	MB index	A measurement of the creatine kinase MB isoenzyme. High levels of CK-MB in the blood may reflect heart muscle damage within 2 to 6 hours of heart attack. *See also:* CK-MB	0–7 ng/mL
	myoglobin	The oxygen-carrying and storage protein of muscle, resembling blood hemoglobin in function; levels are used in the diagnosis of an acute myocardial infarction, as the protein is released into the circulation within 2–4 hours after myocardial infarction, peaks at about 8–12 hours, and returns to normal after 18–24 hours.	<110 ng/mL
	Na	Abbreviation for sodium.	
	natrium	Obsolete term for sodium.	
18	oxygen saturation (SaO_2)	An indication of the relative concentration of hemoglobin in the red blood cells.	97% and higher
	partial pressure of carbon dioxide (PO_2)	Measures the amount of carbon dioxide gas dissolved in the blood. As PCO_2 rises, the blood becomes more acidic.	arterial: 36–46 mmHg venous: 40–52 mmHg

Report #	Term	Definition	Normal Range of Results
	partial pressure of oxygen (PO_2)	Measures the amount of oxygen dissolved in the blood.	arterial: 74–109 mmHg venous: 25–44 mmHg
	partial thromboplastin time activated (PTT, aPTT)	The time needed for plasma to form a fibrin clot following the addition of calcium and a phospholipid reagent; used to evaluate the intrinsic clotting system.	<35 sec
	PCO_2	Abbreviation for partial pressure of carbon dioxide.	
	pH	A symbol indicating hydrogen ion (H+) concentration; scale that measures the relative acidity (0–7.00), alkalinity/basicity (7.00–14.00) and neutrality (6.80) of a solution.	4.6–8.0
4	platelet	A cell fragment that forms a plug to stop bleeding and acts in blood clotting. *Syn:* thrombocyte	
	PO_2	Abbreviation for partial pressure of oxygen.	
4	potassium (K)	An electrolyte that functions to maintain balance of body fluids and is important in nerve and muscle activity.	3.5–5.0 mEq/L
	prostate-specific antigen (PSA)	A glycoprotein found in normal seminal fluid and produced by the prostatic epithelial cells. High levels of PSA are associated with prostate cancer, prostatitis and benign prostatic hyperplasia.	<4.00 ng/mL
	protein	Organic compounds made of amino acids; contains nitrogen, carbon, hydrogen and oxygen and plays a vital role in structures, hormones, enzymes, muscle contraction, immunologic response and essential life functions.	6.0–8.0 g/dL
	prothrombin time (PT)	A test to measure the activity of the protein prothrombin in the blood; measures the time it takes for blood to clot.	9–12 seconds
	PSA	Abbreviation for prostate-specific antigen.	
	PT	Abbreviation for prothrombin time.	
17	pulse oximetry	Used to measure oxygen saturation; performed noninvasively, usually on the finger or ear lobe: the small increase in absorption of light during the systolic pulse is used to calculate oxygen saturation.	*see* oxygen saturation
	RBC, *pl.* RBCs	Abbreviation for red blood cell (count).	

Report #	Term	Definition	Normal Range of Results
	red blood cell count (RBC)	A measurement of red blood cells that transport oxygen bound to hemoglobin throughout the circulatory system.	females: 4.0–5.0 mil/mm^3 males: 4.7–5.7 mil/mm^3
	SaO$_2$	Abbreviation for oxygen saturation.	
4	sodium (Na)	An electrolyte that maintains osmotic balance and body fluid volume.	135–145 mEq/L
	squamous epithelial cells	An abnormal constituent of urine.	positive/negative
	thrombocyte	*Syn:* platelet	
4	troponin	A globular protein that plays a key role in muscle contraction; levels of troponin can become elevated in the blood 3–4 hours after muscle damage occurs following a heart attack.	0.0–0.1 ng/mL
4	UA	Abbreviation for urinalysis.	
4	urinalysis (UA)	Analysis of the urine.	various references
4	WBC	Abbreviation for white blood cell (count).	
11	white blood cell count (WBC)	A measurement of white blood cells which protect against pathogens throughout the circulatory system.	4800–10800/mm^3

Therapeutic Procedures

Invasive, surgical terms

Report #	Term	Definition
29	angioplasty	Reconstitution or recanalization of a blood vessel; may involve balloon dilation, mechanical stripping of intima, forceful injection of fibrinolytics or placement of a stent.
38	aortic valve replacement (AVR)	An open heart procedure to replace the aortic valve with a prosthetic valve due to stenosis or regurgitation.
	aortocoronary bypass	*Syn:* coronary artery bypass graft
44	aortotomy	Incision of the aorta.
27	atriotomy	Incision of an atrium.
	AVR	Abbreviation for aortic valve replacement.
	coronary artery bypass	*Syn:* coronary artery bypass graft
8	CABG	Abbreviation for coronary artery bypass graft; pronounced *cabbage*.

Report #	Term	Definition
27	cardiopulmonary bypass	Diversion of the blood flow returning to the heart through a pump oxygenator (heart-lung machine) and then returning it to the arterial side of the circulation; used in operations upon the heart to maintain extracorporeal circulation.
44	coronary artery bypass graft (CABG)	A conduit, usually a vein graft or internal mammary artery, surgically interposed between the aorta and a coronary artery branch to shunt blood beyond an obstruction. See Figure 26. *Syn:* aortocoronary bypass; coronary artery bypass
	endarterectomy	Excision of atheromatous deposits along with the diseased endothelium and media or most of the media of an artery so as to leave a smooth lining.
44	end-to-side fashion	A suturing technique used to create an anastomosis. The cut end of one structure is sutured to the side of a similar structure. See Figure 27.
	horizontal mattress fashion	A suturing technique in which a double stitch is used to form a loop on both sides of the wound.
	IABP insertion	Abbreviation for intraaortic balloon pump insertion.
	ICD implantation	Abbreviation for implantable cardioverter-defibrillator implantation.

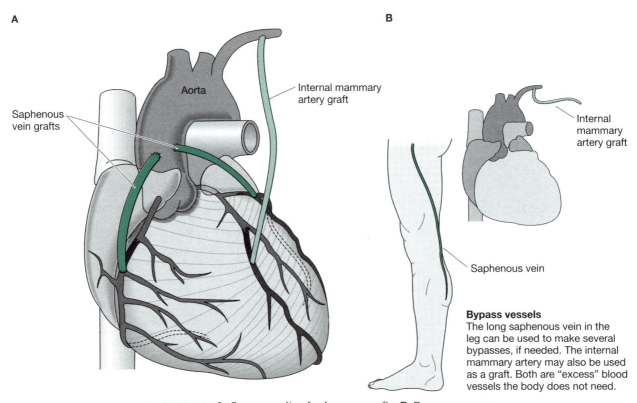

FIGURE 26. A. Common sites for bypass grafts. **B.** Bypass process.

FIGURE 27. Bypass grafting. Grafting is performed under magnification using extremely fine sutures. Each graft is sewn to the aorta, except for the internal mammary artery, which already originates from a branch of the aorta. The other end is sewn to the artery below the blockage.

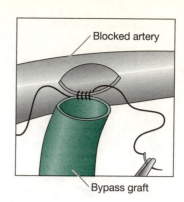

Blocked artery

Bypass graft

Report #	Term	Definition
	implantable cardioverter-defibrillator (ICD) implantation	A pulse generator that may be implanted in the chest, with electrodes attached to the external cardiac surface, or passed through the venous circulation into the right side of the heart. The leads monitor the heart rhythm and send electrical impulses as needed for defibrillation.
48	intraaortic balloon pump (IABP) insertion	An externally actuated and intermittently inflatable balloon that is placed with a catheter into the descending aorta; used to increase blood flow and decrease the heart's workload.
44	midline sternotomy	A vertical incision down the center of the sternum.
	mitral valve replacement (MVR)	An open heart procedure to replace the mitral valve with a prosthetic valve due to stenosis or regurgitation.
	MVR	Abbreviation for mitral valve replacement.
37	pacemaker generator replacement	Replacement of the pulse generator due to battery failure (average lifetime 7–15 years) or other reasons.
41	permanent pacemaker (PPM) implantation	The surgical placement of a pulse generator with attached electrodes or leads. See Figure 2.
	percutaneous coronary intervention	*Syn:* percutaneous transluminal coronary angioplasty
20	percutaneous transluminal coronary angioplasty (PTCA)	An operation to enlarge a narrowed coronary artery by inflating and withdrawing a balloon on the tip of an angiographic catheter. See Figure 28. *Syn:* percutaneous coronary intervention
	PPM implantation	Abbreviation for permanent pacemaker implantation.
2	PTCA	Abbreviation for percutaneous transluminal coronary angioplasty.
48	surgical revascularization	Reestablishment of blood supply to a body part by surgical intervention.

Predilation angiogram revealing 99% stenosis of the right coronary artery (RCA).

PTCA procedure showing catheter placement and straddling of the balloon at the occluded site.

Post-PTCA angiogram showing successful dilation.

Wall of coronary artery

Plaque

Catheter in place; balloon deflated

Balloon inflated

Plaque expanded; catheter removed

Dashed lines indicate old plaque thickness

FIGURE 28. Percutaneous transluminal coronary angioplasty (PTCA).

Report #	Term	Definition
48, 49	temporary transvenous pacemaker wire insertion	A temporary implantation of a pacemaker lead or electrode through a vein into the heart to relieve symptoms; may precede permanent pacemaker implantation.
	topical hypothermia using iced slush solution	Procedure done during open heart surgery to cool the heart using an iced slush solution.
44	venotomy	Incision into a vein.

Noninvasive terms

Report #	Term	Definition
	cardiopulmonary resuscitation (CPR)	Restoration of cardiac output and pulmonary ventilation following cardiac arrest and apnea, using artificial respiration and manual closed-chest compression or open-chest cardiac massage.
38	cardioversion	Restoration of the heart's rhythm to normal by electrical countershock or by medications.
2	CPR	Abbreviation for cardiopulmonary resuscitation.
50	defibrillation threshold testing	Testing the point at which a stimulus first produces a response in an implantable defibrillator.
50	programming	Setting the parameters of a pulse generator for pacing mode, sensitivity, rate and other programmable features.

Therapeutic Drugs and Medications Commonly Used in Cardiology

Medications by generic name

Report #	Generic Name	Drug Class	Route of Administration	Definition
	acetylsalicylic acid (ASA)	antiplatelet agent, analgesic	caplet, tablet	*Syn:* aspirin
	adenosine	antiarrhythmic	injection	For treatment of paroxysmal supraventricular tachycardia. Also used instead of exercise to stress the heart during stress studies.
15	amiodarone	antiarrhythmic	injection, tablet	For treatment of ventricular tachycardia and ventricular fibrillation.
11	ASA	antiplatelet agent, analgesic	caplet, tablet	Abbreviation for acetylsalicylic acid. *Syn:* aspirin
11	aspirin	antiplatelet agent, analgesic	caplet, tablet	For treatment of mild to moderate pain, inflammation and fever; prophylaxis of myocardial infarction and other uses. *Syn:* acetylsalicylic acid
	atenolol	beta-adrenergic blocker	injection, tablet	For treatment of hypertension, management of angina pectoris and postmyocardial infarction.
	atorvastatin	HMG-CoA reductase inhibitor	tablet	For primary prevention of cardiovascular disease by reducing cholesterol levels.
	calcium; calcium replete	mineral supplement	capsule, tablet	Mineral supplement to replenish calcium levels necessary in muscle contraction, blood clotting and other functions.
	captopril	ACE inhibitor	tablet	For management of hypertension.
	cardioplegic solution	organ preservation solution	injection	A solution to paralyze the heart and preserve myocardial metabolism during open-heart surgery.
	carvedilol	beta-adrenergic blocker	tablet	For treatment in mild to severe heart failure and left ventricular dysfunction.

Report #	Generic Name	Drug Class	Route of Administration	Definition
	cefazolin	cephalosporin	infusion, injection	For treatment of respiratory, skin, bone, joint and blood infections. Commonly administered intraoperatively to protect against infection.
	clopidogrel	antiplatelet agent	tablet (film coated)	For reducing atherosclerotic events such as myocardial infarction, stroke and other vascular deaths.
15	digoxin	antiarrhythmic	injection	For treatment of congestive heart failure and to slow ventricular rate in tachyarrhythmias.
	diltiazem	calcium channel blocker	capsule, injection, tablet	For treatment of angina, hypertension, paroxysmal supraventricular tachycardia, atrial fibrillation and atrial flutter.
12	dipyridamole	antiplatelet agent	injection, tablet	Used with warfarin to decrease thrombosis after valve replacement and as a diagnostic agent in coronary artery disease.
27	dopamine	adrenergic agonist agent	infusion, injection	For treatment of shock (e.g., myocardial infarction, open heart surgery, renal failure).
	enteric coated aspirin	antiplatelet agent, analgesic	tablet	Aspirin that is coated with a material to prevent or minimize dissolution in the stomach but allows dissolution in the small intestine. This type of formulation protects the stomach from potential irritation.
30	epinephrine	adrenergic agonist agent	aerosol or oral inhalation, injection, solution for oral inhalation	For treatment of cardiac arrest, bronchospasms; also added to anesthetics and other agents.
	epoetin alfa	colony-stimulating factor	injection	For treatment of anemia.
	eptifibatide	antiplatelet agent	injection	For treatment of acute coronary syndrome.

Report #	Generic Name	Drug Class	Route of Administration	Definition
25	fentanyl	analgesic, narcotic	infusion, injection, lozenge, transdermal system (Duragesic)	For sedation and pain relief.
	furosemide	diuretic	injection, solution (oral), tablet (Lasix)	For management of edema.
9	heparin; IV heparin	anticoagulant	infusion, injection	For prophylaxis and treatment of clotting disorders.
21	lidocaine	analgesic, antiarrhythmic	topical, injection	For acute treatment of ventricular arrhythmias from myocardial infarction; also used as an anesthetic as well as other purposes.
11	lisinopril	ACE inhibitor	tablet	For treatment of hypertension, acute MI, etc.
	magnesium	mineral supplement	capsule, tablet	A mineral supplement for cell processes.
	metoprolol	beta-adrenergic blocker	injection, tablet	For treatment of hypertension and angina pectoris, prevention of MI and other disorders.
	midazolam	benzodiazepine	injection, syrup	Provides preoperative sedation and conscious sedation before diagnostic procedures.
	morphine; morphine sulfate	analgesic, narcotic	capsule, injection, solution (oral), suppository, tablet	For relief in moderate to severe pain, dyspnea in CHF and as a preanesthetic.
15	nitroglycerin	vasodilator	capsule, infusion, injection, ointment, solution, tablet, transdermal system	For treatment of angina pectoris.
	potassium; replete potassium	mineral supplement	injection, tablet, capsule, infusion, powder (oral), solution (oral)	A mineral supplement necessary for fluid balance and muscle and nerve activity.
	povidone-iodine	antibacterial	gel (topical), liquid (topical), liquid scrub, ointment, solution, swab sticks	An external antiseptic to kill bacteria, fungi, viruses, protozoa and yeasts.

Report #	Generic Name	Drug Class	Route of Administration	Definition
50	procainamide	antiarrhythmic	capsule, injection, tablet	For treatment of ventricular tachycardia, paroxysmal supraventricular tachycardia, premature ventricular contraction and atrial fibrillation.
	propofol	general anesthesia	injection	For sedation and anesthesia.
27	protamine	antidote	injection	For neutralizing heparin during surgery.
	sodium polystyrene sulfonate	antidote	powder (oral/rectal), suspension (oral/rectal)	For treatment of hyperkalemia.
9	spironolactone	diuretic	tablet	For management of edema.
	warfarin	anticoagulant	injection, tablet	For prophylaxis and treatment of venous thrombosis, pulmonary embolism and clotting disorders.

Medications by brand name

Report #	Brand Name	Generic Name
	Adenocard	adenosine
	Adenoscan	adenosine
	Adrenalin Chloride	epinephrine
	Aldactazide	spironolactone
	Aldactone	spironolactone
25	Ancef	cefazolin
	Aspergum	aspirin
	Asprimox	aspirin
	Astramorph PF	morphine
	Avinza	morphine
	Bayer	aspirin
26	Betadine	povidone-iodine
	Capoten	captopril
	Cardizem; Cardizem CD; Cardizem LA	diltiazem

Report #	Brand Name	Generic Name
	Cartia XT	diltiazem
	Cordarone	amiodarone
15	Coreg	carvedilol
13	Coumadin	warfarin
	Darvon Compound 32	aspirin
	DepoDur	morphine
45	Digitek	digoxin
	Dilacor XR	diltiazem
	Diltia XT	diltiazem
	Dilt-XR	diltiazem
38	Diprivan	propofol
	Duragesic	fentanyl
	Duramorph	morphine
	Easprin	aspirin
	Ecotrin	enteric coated aspirin
	EpiPen; EpiPen Jr.	epinephrine
	Epogen	epoetin alfa
	Genprin	aspirin
	Halfprin 81	aspirin
	Heartline	aspirin
	Hepflush-10	heparin
	Hep-Lock; Hep-Lock U/P	heparin
	Humalog Mix 50/50; Humalog Mix 75/25	protamine
	Infumorph 200; Infumorph 500	morphine
48	Integrilin	eptifibatide
	Intropin	dopamine
	Jantoven	warfarin
	Kadian	morphine
	Kayexalate	sodium polystyrene sulfonate
	Lanoxicaps	digoxin
	Lanoxin	digoxin

Report #	Brand Name	Generic Name
9	Lasix	furosemide
	Lipitor	atorvastatin
	Lipo-Hepin; Lipo-Hepin/BL	heparin
	Liquaemin	heparin
13	Lopressor	metoprolol
	MD Contin	morphine
	microNefrin	epinephrine
	Minitran	nitroglycerin
	Niglycon	nitroglycerin
	Niong	nitroglycerin
	Nitrek	nitroglycerin
	Nitro-Bid	nitroglycerin
	Nitrocels	nitroglycerin
	Nitrodisc	nitroglycerin
	Nitro-Dur	nitroglycerin
	Nitrodyl	nitroglycerin
	Nitrogard	nitroglycerin
	Nitrolingual	nitroglycerin
	Nitro-Lyn	nitroglycerin
	NitroQuick	nitroglycerin
	Nitrospan	nitroglycerin
	Nitrostat	nitroglycerin
	NitroTab	nitroglycerin
	Nitro-Time	nitroglycerin
	Norwich Aspirin	aspirin
	Oramorph SR	morphine
	Pacerone	amiodarone
12	Persantine; Persantine IV	dipyridamole
9	Plavix	clopidogrel
	Plegisol	cardioplegic solution
	Prinivil	lisinopril
	Procanbid	procainamide

Report #	Brand Name	Generic Name
	Procrit	epoetin alfa
	Roxanol; Roxanol 100; Roxanol T	morphine
	St. Joseph	aspirin
	Taztia XT	diltiazem
	Tenormin	atenolol
	Tiamate	diltiazem
	Tiazac; Tiazac ER	diltiazem
	Transderm-Nitro	nitroglycerin
17	Versed	midazolam
25	Xylocaine	lidocaine
	Zestril	lisinopril
	Zilactin-L	lidocaine
	Zolicef	cefazolin
	ZORprin	aspirin

Equipment and Instrumentation

Report #	Term	Definition
	#10, #11, #12, #15 blade; *var.* 10-blade, 11-blade, 12-blade, 15-blade	A scalpel blade of a specific size.
	4 x 4 gauze	A gauze or bandage four inches square.
	active-fixation lead	A pacemaker electrode designed with a metal screw-in device to affix itself into the endocardial lining.
	Adler retractor	A proprietary instrument for drawing aside the edges of a wound or for holding back structures adjacent to the operative field.
37	Affinity SR pulse generator	A brand name pacemaker generator by Pacesetter, Inc.
	anchoring sleeve	A device to facilitate insertion and fixation of a pacemaker lead.
	aortic cannulation device	A tube that can be inserted into the aorta as a channel for the transport of fluid.
	Argon needle	Surgical tool from Argon Medical Devices; various sizes used in cardiologic surgery and exploration.

Report #	Term	Definition
30	Arrow introducer sheath	A brand name for a specially designed tubular instrument introduced transvenously and through which surgical instruments can be passed.
28	Bovie cautery	An instrument used for electrosurgical dissection and hemostasis. Frequently used as a verb, i.e., to Bovie something is to dissect or cauterize it with the Bovie instrument.
44	bulldog clamps	A specially designed surgical instrument for compression or holding a structure.
8	cannula	A tube that can be inserted into a cavity or vein, usually by means of a trocar filling its lumen; after the insertion of the cannula, the trocar is withdrawn and the cannula remains as a channel for the transport of fluid.
	Carbomedics valve	A brand name prosthetic valve.
44	chest tube	A tube placed through the chest wall that drains the pleural space.
50	CPI Mini IV transvenous defibrillator	*Syn:* Guidant Ventak Mini IV
42	dilator	An instrument designed for enlarging a hollow structure or opening.
	electrocautery	An instrument for directing a high-frequency current through a local area of tissue for hemostasis or dissection.
	endocardial pacing electrode	A pacemaker lead that is affixed into the innermost layer of the heart.
	epicardial electrode	A pacemaker lead placed on the exterior heart tissue.
27	Ethibond suture	A suture made out of a specific proprietary material.
44	figure-of-eight suture	A suture using criss-cross stitches to approximate fascial edges or the musculofascial and outer layers of an abdominal wound.
	Foley catheter	A urethral catheter with a retaining balloon.
5	French	A scale for grading sizes of sounds, tubes and catheters; a diameter of 1/3 mm equals 1 French.
	fresh frozen plasma	Separated plasma, frozen within 6 hours of collection, used in cases of hypovolemia and coagulation factor deficiency.
50	Guidant Ventak Mini IV	A brand name implantable cardioverter-defibrillator generator. *Syn:* CPI Mini IV transvenous defibrillator
26	guidewire, *var.* guide wire	A wire or spring used as a guide for placement of a larger device or prosthesis such as a catheter or intramedullary pin.
	Halsted suture	*Syn:* subcuticular suture
43	Hemaquet	Proprietary device made by USCI used to introduce catheters transdermally. Some sizes of Hemaquet devices were recalled in 1993.

Report #	Term	Definition
	Integrity AFXDR pulse generator	A brand name pacemaker generator manufactured by Pacesetter, Inc.
	Intermedics single-coil defibrillator	A brand name defibrillator electrode placed into the endocardium.
21	JL4	Abbreviation for Judkins left (catheter); the number indicates the type of curve.
21	JR4	Abbreviation for Judkins right (catheter); the number indicates the type of curve.
	Judkins catheter	A catheter of a specific shape used in coronary angiography. A Judkins right catheter is used in the right coronary artery; a Judkins left catheter is used in the left coronary artery.
	large-bore needle	Refers to the greater size of the lumen of the needle.
28	Medtronic atrial lead, screw-in model	A brand name pacemaker electrode placed into the atrium.
15	Medtronic bipolar endocardial lead	A brand name pacemaker electrode placed into the endocardium.
	Medtronic Gem II DR automatic implantable defibrillator	A brand name dual-chamber rate-responsive implantable defibrillator.
	Medtronic pulse generator Kappa DR	A brand name dual-chamber implantable pulse generator.
28	Medtronic Sprint ventricular lead	A brand name pacemaker electrode placed into the ventricle.
	nebulizer	A device used to reduce liquid medication to extremely fine cloud-like particles; useful in delivering medication to deeper parts of the respiratory tract.
	NIR with Sox stent	A specific type of stent; inserts a mesh tube into a diseased artery to hold it open.
	normal saline	A sterile solution containing water and sodium chloride.
	pacemaker lead	A wire that transmits impulses from an artificial pacemaker to the heart.
37	pacemaker pocket	A pouch-like cavity where the pacemaker pulse generator is placed.
48	pacemaker wire	An electrode or lead attached to a pulse generator.
37	pacer site	The location of the pacemaker generator.
	Pacesetter atrial lead	A brand name pacemaker electrode placed into the atrium.
	Pacesetter ventricular lead	A brand name pacemaker electrode placed into the ventricle.
	Patriot wire	A peripheral guidewire used during angiography.

Report #	Term	Definition
5, 46	pigtail catheter	A catheter with a tightly curled end and multiple side holes to reduce the impact of the injectant on the vessel wall or to remain in a chamber or space for drainage.
44	pledgeted stitch	A suture supported by a small piece of fabric or tissue so that the suture will not tear through the tissue.
15	pressure dressing	A dressing by which pressure is exerted on the area covered to prevent the collection of fluids in the underlying tissues.
17	probe	A slender rod of rigid or flexible material with a blunt bulbous tip, used for exploring.
27	Prolene suture	A brand name synthetic coating on nonabsorbable suture material.
	prosthetic valve	An artificial valve used to replace a human valve.
	prosthetic valve leaflet	A thin flattened object or structure associated with the reduplication of heart valve tissue.
44	pulmonary artery catheter	A tubular instrument to allow passage of fluid into or out of the pulmonary artery.
37	pulse generator	A device that produces an electrical discharge through an attached electrode into the heart muscle to produce a contraction. *Syn:* pacemaker
	Ranger balloon	A specific type of brand name balloon catheter.
27	retractor	An instrument for drawing aside and holding back structures.
43	right coronary catheter	A tubular instrument used to allow passage of fluid into or out of the right coronary artery.
5	sheath	A specially designed tubular instrument through which special obturators or cutting instruments can be passed, or through which blood clots, tissue fragments and calculi can be evacuated (i.e., balloon pump sheath, arterial sheath, introducer sheath).
28	silk	Material used as a suture.
	skin staple	A piece of stainless steel wire used by a stapling device that unites layers of tissue.
	snare	An instrument for removing polyps and other projections from a surface, especially within a cavity; it consists of a wire loop that is passed around the base of the mass and then gradually tightened.
30	stainless steel wires	Wire sutures used to fasten ends of tissue together; typically used to suture bony structures such as the sternum.
49	Steri-Strips	A brand name for a type of self-adhesive bandage.
	sternal retractor	An instrument for drawing aside and for holding back the sternum and adjacent structures to the operative field.
	sternal saw	A metal operating instrument having an edge of sharp, toothlike projections for cutting the sternum.

Report #	Term	Definition
27	sternal wires	Steel wires used for sternal closure after open heart surgery.
44	subcuticular suture	A suture placed through the subcuticular fascia; used for exact skin approximation. *Syn:* Halsted suture
	Telfa dressing	A cotton dressing enclosed in perforated plastic to prevent adherence to the wound.
	transesophageal probe	A slender rod of rigid or flexible material, with a blunt bulbous tip, used for exploring the esophagus.
49	transvenous balloon-type catheter	A catheter used in arterial embolectomy or to float into the pulmonary artery.
49	transvenous temporary pacemaker	Temporary insertion of a pacemaker lead or electrode through a vein into the heart to regulate the heart rhythm and rate.
25	VasoSeal	A brand name arterial puncture sealing product that provides hemostasis.
30	venous cannula	Tube for insertion into a vessel for fluid transport.
	ventricular electrode	A pacemaker lead designed for placement in the lower heart chamber. *Syn:* ventricular lead
28	ventricular lead	*Syn:* ventricular electrode
28	Vicryl	A brand name synthetic coating on absorbable suture material.

COMMON CARDIOVASCULAR PHRASES

Report #	Phrase	Report #	Phrase
	acute ischemic event	44	atrial pacing wires
40	adequate excursion		blood pressure response is physiologic
26, 41	advanced using fluoroscopic guidance	43	brisk filling
	age predicted maximum (heart rate)	33	burst atrial pacing
	aneurysmal dilatation	2	cardiac catheterization lab
	angiography suite	15	carotid bruits
16	anicteric sclera	16	carotid upstrokes not delayed
1	antegrade flow	43	catheter engagement
40	appeared grossly normal	2	catheterization lab
	arrhythmic events	4	chief complaint
	atherosclerotic calcifications	13	chronic anticoagulation
30	atrial cannula	27	coaptation of the leaflets

Report #	Phrase
44	cold cardioplegia
17	color flow
43	competitive spilling
43	concentric distal narrowing
4	conjunctivae clear
	constellation of symptoms
48	continuous pressure monitoring
27	cooling to 28 degrees
30	crystalloid cardioplegia
44	decent lumen
	decorticate with ventilatory respirations
50	defibrillator pocket
	detach detection rate
	detection rate limit
23	diastolic noncompliance
48	diffuse disease
43	diffuse irregularity
	discharged to home
16	discomfort with inspiration
	discrete lesion
43	distal narrowing
	distal pulses
48	dominant vessel
	drawback pressure was obtained
	ductal level
40	E:A ratio
48	eccentric stenosis
9	edema of +2
12	ECG changes
28	electrophysiology laboratory
21, 43, 48	end-diastolic pressure
50	endocardial anchoring

Report #	Phrase
8	episodic angina
	evidence of ectasia
	exercise-induced chest pain
	extravascular dye staining was noted
43	fair-caliber vessel
	fixed decreased uptake
28	fluoroscopic guidance
	flushed and irrigated
	flushed with normal saline
	found to be stable
	free of focal stenosis
5	free of significant plaque
50	free-form pocket
30, 43, 48	gives rise to
39, 43	global hypokinesis
	globally preserved
40	global wall motion abnormalities
44	good quality vein
	greatly modified protocol
6	grossly normal
	gross blood was aspirated
	guidewire was inserted, guidewire was placed
16	heart sounds are regular without gallops or murmurs
4	history and physical (H&P)
44	hood of the PDA graft
44	hot cardioplegia
	hot shot of blood cardioplegia
26, 41	in a fasting state
22	in the usual manner
21	informed consent was obtained
	injection system

Report #	Phrase
44	inotropic support
	INR is therapeutic
	interrogation of the valves
	intimal thickening
	intraoperative electrophysiologic study
49	intravenous fluid was infused
	irregular heartbeat
	irregular segmental stenosis
24, 27, 30	irrigated with antibiotic-saline solution
	jugular venous pressure (JVP)
48	large-caliber vessel
28	lead was actively fixed
	limb leads
48	limbs of the bifurcation
40	low cardiac output
15	lower extremity edema
13	lungs were clear to auscultation
44	lungs were inflated
7 14	maximal heart rate; maximum heart rate
	mid epigastric area
48	mild diffuse disease
40	moderately dilated
40	moderately enlarged
	modest-sized vessel
	near syncopal
4	no acute distress (NAD)
14	no arrhythmias noted
3	no complications
12	no ECG changes
9, 21	nonischemic cardiomyopathy
	nonocclusive dissection

Report #	Phrase
	nonspecific complaints
	nonspecific ST-segment changes
	normal axis
6	normal dimension
	normal in caliber
	normalization at rest
43	obstructive disease
43	obstructive lesions
26, 50	over a guidewire
	pacing and sensing parameters were obtained
44	packed with ice
	palpable pulse
4	patient denies
3	patient tolerated the procedure well
	patient was alert and oriented
44	patient was heparinized
44	patient was rewarmed
44	patient was ventilated
22	peak heart rate
	pharmacological study
44	plaque emanating
25	poor candidate for anticoagulation therapy
	poor exercise tolerance
	posterolateral branches
	posterior tibial pulsations
	predicted age-adjusted maximum heart rate
43	premedications administered
8	prepped and draped in a sterile manner; prepped and draped in the usual sterile fashion
23, 34	preserved left ventricular function
	principal marginal

Report #	Phrase	Report #	Phrase
	presented to the hospital		telemetry unit
	pulse generator pocket	48	testing of thresholds
	pulse oximetry on room air	50	threshold testing via the pacing system analyzer ensued
	pulses were intact but weakened		trace edema
	pupils normal and reactive to light		transaortic gradient
44	pursestring was ligated	49	triangle between the medial and lateral heads of the trapezius muscles
	rales and rhonchi		
50	reliably induced ventricular fibrillation	28	under fluoroscopic guidance
4	respirations even and unlabored	9	unremarkable
44	reverse saphenous vein	40	upper limits of normal
16	risk factors		uptake of Tc-99m sestamibi
	risk/benefit ratio		urine sample
	risks and benefits		vascular access
	saturating 100% on 2 liters oxygen via nasal cannula		veins were compressible
			velocity measurements
23	sclerotic changes		ventricular cavity dilatation
4	shortness of breath (SOB)		ventricular contractility
44	single-clamp technique	44	ventricular pacing wires
	single-wall puncture	44	ventricular vent
44	small serial incisions with skin bridges		ventricle was de-aired
	source of emboli		vesicular breath sounds
	spontaneous echo contrast	49	via the side ports of the catheter
27, 30	spontaneous sinus rhythm		visually estimated
2	status post (S/P; SP)	44	volume status was normalized
	structurally normal-appearing	6	wall motion
	submaximal stress test		wall thickening
40	suboptimally imaged	44	weaned off bypass
6	systolic function		weight-adjusted dose
28	tear-away sheath	1	widely patent
	teased off (from the diaphragm or another structure)	5	with no evidence
	technically difficult to visualize		within acceptable ranges
40	technically adequate study	4	within normal limits
		21	without complications

part 2

Medical Transcription Practice

The key to growing one's transcription proficiency is through practice. Nothing can replace the value gained by listening to physician dictation and transcribing what has been dictated. To that end, the CD-ROM found in the back of this book contains 50 dictated reports in the field of cardiology, along with corresponding Answer Keys. The reports range in complexity from easiest to most difficult. Each Answer Key is available as a PDF file, which not only displays the final transcribed report, but has also been carefully reviewed to provide valuable feedback on the various components of the report, to point out challenges specific to the dictation and to indicate common stumbling blocks encountered when transcribing these types of reports. Where applicable, sources for grammar, style and usage rules have been incorporated into the PDF Answer Keys.

Each Answer Key is also available as a Microsoft Word file. Please note that the MS Word files do not include feedback, so it is recommended that you review the PDF file when comparing your transcribed report to an Answer Key. The MS Word files are particularly useful in the classroom or for electronically comparing your transcript to the Answer Key.

When transcribing the reports, use a report format (headings, spacing, etc.) with which you are familiar, or use the format that is required by your facility. Note that the formatting you use in your report will probably not match what appears in the Answer Key, but this is acceptable as long as you remain consistent with your heading styles.

To access the Medical Transcription Practice Audio Dictation Files and Answer Keys, install the *Creating Cardiology Reports* CD-ROM to your computer following the steps found on p. 1 of this workbook.

To open *Stedman's Medical Transcription Skill Builders: Creating Cardiology Reports*:

1. From the Start menu, select Programs.

2. From the Programs menu, select the Stedman's program group.

3. From the Stedman's program group, select *MT Skill Builders Cardiology*.

Refer to the Help Files for detailed information on how to use the program.

Using Your Foot Pedal with Stedman's Medical Transcription Skill Builders Audio Dictation Files

The Medical Transcription Practice Audio Files are designed to play through your default wav player. This feature allows you to play and transcribe the reports using the program of your choice rather than requiring you to play the files through an audio player built into the *Stedman's Medical Transcription Skill Builders* program.

If the program you wish to use to play the *Stedman's* audio dictation files does not launch when you open an audio file from the *Stedman's Medical Transcription Skill Builders* menu, you will need to change your default wav player settings.

To learn how to change your default settings, please refer to the User's Guide or Help Files that came with your audio player or foot pedal. Alternatively, you can follow these instructions to modify your default wav player settings:

1. Locate any wav file on your hard drive, right-click on it and choose **Open With. . .**

2. Scroll through the list of programs to locate your preferred audio player or foot pedal program *or* choose **Browse...** and locate the EXE file for your audio player or foot pedal.

3. Select the box that says **Always use the selected program to open this kind of file** and click **OK**.

Once you have modified your default wav player settings, return to the *Stedman's Medical Transcription Skill Builders* menu and choose one of the audio dictation files. The program you selected in the steps above will be used to play the audio dictation file.

Terminology and Abbreviations Used in the Medical Transcription Practice Answer Keys

The abbreviations and terms below are used throughout the PDF Answer Keys to succinctly provide feedback and remediation.

Feedback	Meaning
alt.	acceptable alternative
facility	the hospital, clinic, medical transcription company or other organization or business for which the report is being transcribed (i.e., your employer)
note	helpful information that does not necessitate a change to the report
organization	the hospital, clinic, medical transcription company or other organization or business for which the report is being transcribed (i.e., your employer)
originator	the person who is dictating the report; also called the author or dictator
preferable	indicates a style, grammar or usage directive for which AAMT states a preference but does not assert as a "rule"
s/b	"should be"
spell out, write out	write out the full term instead of using an abbreviation or symbol

Sources for Grammar, Style and Usage Rules	Refers To
AAMT Book of Style	The AAMT Book of Style for Medical Transcription, 2nd Edition
AMA Manual of Style	American Medical Association Manual of Style, 9th Edition
ISMP	The Institute for Safe Medication Practices
JCAHO	Joint Commission on the Accreditation of Healthcare Organizations
Merriam-Webster Online	Merriam-Webster Online Dictionary, www.m-w.com
Stedman's Medical Dictionary, 28E	Stedman's Medical Dictionary, 28th Edition

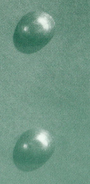

part 3

Proofreading and Editing Exercises

Editing and proofreading have become crucial aspects of document refinement due to the increasing significance of accurate medical documentation for patient care, the need to request appropriate reimbursement, and the resolution of medical malpractice suits. As a result, the call for experienced quality assurance (QA) personnel is rapidly evolving into an alternative career for many medical transcriptionists.

The evolution of cardiac medicine, coupled with a greater need for QA, has prompted a push for development and refinement of QA skills within the medical transcription industry.

The sample reports contained in this section are an important resource for those wishing to learn or improve the skills necessary to achieve excellence in the processes of editing and proofreading.

The Quality Assurance Process

The process of QA is similar to medical transcription in that it begins with the careful selection of reference materials, such as a style guide, proofreading guidelines, English and medical dictionaries, and other resources necessary to confirm that final determinations are accurate. Those engaged in QA should be familiar with abbreviations and acronyms that are no longer acceptable and with current HIPAA regulations. These items directly contribute to patient safety and privacy.

When reviewing cardiology reports for QA, it helps to be familiar with common dictation errors. For example, P wave is often dictated instead of R wave (in the ventricle); aortic pressure value is given when left ventricular pressure is meant; and the mitral valve is stated as having three leaflets when they should be associated with the aortic valve.

Take the time to learn the normal parameters for common measurements given during echocardiography and catheterization dictation. The cardiologist routinely dictates name brands, named protocols and national studies (i.e., MADIT II), so it is important to keep references as current as possible.

Report Formats

To reflect the diversity of formats used in the process of medical documentation, the reports in this section include an assortment of layouts and heading names. These are meant to showcase the different report structures transcriptionists will encounter on the job; however, transcriptionists are urged to familiarize themselves with and should always follow the guidelines set by their employers.

How to Complete the Proofreading and Editing Exercises

Each sample report is designed to challenge your skill set, whether you are just starting out or if you've been transcribing cardiology reports for awhile. When a change is necessary, use standard proofreaders' marks (see Appendix A) to ensure consistency in making corrections. These marks can also be found in most English dictionaries.

Once a change has been marked, include a very brief note that identifies the source to verify the necessity or accuracy of the change. This practice lends credibility to the process and provides an explanation to the medical transcriptionist who is responsible for changing the document.

After you have completed the Exercise, refer to the corresponding Answer Key and For Signature (or *Final*) report for remediation. The Answer Keys begin on page 147. The edits that you see in the Answer Keys were made with the goal of creating a document that is clear and in accordance with the rules and recommendations found in the AAMT Book of Style, 2nd Edition. Understand that every facility has its own policies and requirements, so some of the edits contained in the Answer Keys may not be applicable to the hospital or clinic for which you work. For example, some facilities forbid the transcriptionist to make any modifications to sentence structure;

some do not allow for paragraph breaks. In addition, dictation systems often impose their own limitations on how reports appear. Numbered lists may need to be formatted in a very specific way, and unusual formats or characters, such as subscript superscript formatting, may be stripped out by the dictation system. Again, we advise you to acquaint yourself with the rules and regulations of your facility and to incorporate these in your proofreading and editing.

Sample reports have always provided an effective guide for finding new or difficult terms and have served as a true representation of transcription. The sample reports contained in this section are sure to continue that tradition and become a valuable resource for medical transcriptionists and for those engaged in quality assurance programs.

Proofreading & Editing Exercise

Report #1

CAROTID DUPLEX SCAN

CAROTID IMAGING

NAME OF TEST: Carotid duplex scan.

INDICATIONS: The patient is a 77 year old man with a known occlusion of the right internal carotid artery and a left carotid artery bypass.

RIGHT CAROTID ARTERY: The internal carotid is occluded. The common and external carotid arteries are widely patent.

LEFT CAROTID ARTERY: The bypass graft from the common to the internal carotid is widely patent. The external carotid appears to be occluded.

VERTEBRAL FLOW: Antegrade on the right and auscultatory on the left.

IMPRESSION:

Occlusion of the right internal carotid artery. Widely patent left carotid bypass. Auscultatory flow in the left vertebral artery is suggestive a left subclavian steel syndrome.

Proofreading & Editing Exercise

Report #2

DEATH SUMMARY

CLINICAL RESUME

FINAL DIAGNOSIS:

1. Status post acute anterior wall myocardial infarction with left ventricular aneurysm.
2. Ischemic cardiomyopathy.

HOSPITAL COURSE: This was an 87-year-old lady who was visiting this area, presently to the emergency room with symptoms of acute unstable angina. She was noted to have ST-segment elevation in the inferior and anterior leads. She was brought urgently to the cardiac catheterization lab where angiography revealed total occlusion of the mid left anterior descending artery, which appeared to be an old occlusion. The right coronary artery had a 99% proximal stenosis. The left ventriculogram revealed several anteroapical hypokinesia with an aneurysm of the apex of the left ventricle. Since she was having ongoing pain, she underwent PTCA and stenting of the left coronary artery. A 3.0 x 33 cm Cypher stent was deployed with a good result. The patient did very well subsequently. However, on the date of her demise at around 12:30, the patient collapsed on her bed. She was noted to initially be in ventricular fibrillation. She was defibrillated, then she went into pulseless electrical activity despite CPR for a prolonged period time. She could not be resuscitated and was pronounced dead.

Proofreading & Editing Exercise

PSEUDOANEURYSM THROMBIN INJECTION

CARDIOVASCULAR PROCEDURE REPORT

PROCEDURE: Right groin thrombin injection under ultrasound guidance.

PREPROCEDURE AND POSTPROCEDURE DIAGNOSIS: Right groin pseudoaneurysm.

INDICATION: This is a 72-year-old female with a significant past medical history of a right groin pseudoaneurysm after a heart catheterization.

FINDINGS: She has a right groin pseudoaneurysm that was successfully thrombosed.

PROCEDURE: After informed written consent was obtained, the patient was placed in a supine position. The right groin was prepped and draped and, using a spinal needle, a direct thrombin injection was performed using 3000-4000 units of thrombin into the pseudoaneurysm. This abruptly occluded the pseudoaneurysm. The patient tolerated the procedure well. The patient was sent to recovery area in good condition. There were no complications.

Proofreading & Editing Exercise

HISTORY AND PHYSICAL EXAMINATION FOR CHEST PAIN

HISTORY AND PHYSICAL EXAMINATION

CHIEF COMPLAINT: Chest pain.

HISTORY OF PRESENT ILLNESS: The patient is a 47-year-old female with a history of hypertension, gastroesophageal reflux disease, who presented to the emergency room with complaints of intermittent mid-sternal chest pain that has been ongoing for the past three weeks. Patient reports that her pain was worse this morning, with radiation to her back and associated shortness of breath. Patient also has a history of hypertension and has been off her medications for the past two weeks. She denies any associated dyspnea on exertion, fever, chills, weakness, palpitations, diaphoresis, cough, nausea, vomiting, orthopnea, congestion, or any other systems at this time. Electrocardiogram revealed normal sinus rhythm. Initial troponin was noted to be 0.01.

PAST MEDICAL HISTORY: Hypertension, gastroesophageal reflux disease, iron deficiency anemia secondary to menorrhagia.

PAST SURGICAL HISTORY: Bilateral tubal ligation.

SOCIAL HISTORY: Patient denies any alcohol, tobacco, or illicit drug use.

FAMILY HISTORY: Noncontributory.

REVIEW OF SYSTEMS: General: Patient denies fever, chills, weight loss or weakness. Cardiovascular/respiratory: As noted in HPI. GI: Denies nausea, vomiting, diarrhea, abdominal pain, GI bleed. Neurologic: Denies headache, loss of consciousness, syncope, near syncope. Musculoskeletal: Denies joint swelling, neck pain, back pain. Eyes: Denies visual changes or pain. ENT: Denies sore throat, earache, hearing changes. Hematology: Patient has a history of iron deficiency anemia secondary to menorrhagia. Dermatology: Denies rash, pruritis, laceration, or contusion. Psychiatric: Denies depression, anxiety, suicidal or homicidal delusion or ideation. GU: Positive for urinary frequency. Denies dysuria or hematuria, vaginal discharge or bleed. Endocrine: Denies heat or cold intolerance, thyroid trouble.

PHYSICAL EXAMINATION: VITAL SIGNS: Blood pressure 211/105, respirations 20, pulse 65, temperature 98.4. GENERAL: A well-developed, well-nourished 47-year-old female in no acute distress. HEENT: Normocephalic, without lesions. Sclerae, conjunctivae clear. Extraocular movements are intact. Pupils equal and reactive to light. Oropharynx within normal limits. NECK: Supple, with full range of motion. No lymphadenopathy, JVD, or bruits noted. CARDIAC: Normal S1, S2 without murmurs, gallops, or clicks present. LUNGS: Respirations even and unlabored. Lung fields without wheezes, rales, or rhonchi. CHEST: Mid-sternal epigastric tenderness noted

(continued)

on presentation. ABDOMEN: Soft with mild epigastric tenderness. Bowel sounds present. Liver, spleen, and kidneys not palpable. GENITOURINARY: Deferred. PELVIC/RECTAL: Deferred. EXTREMITIES: Symmetrical, without cyanosis, clubbing, edema, or varicosities. Normal range of motion of extremities noted. NEUROLOGIC: Cranial nerves 2 through 12 grossly intact. No sensory or motor deficit. INTEGUMENTARY: No open areas or lesions noted. MENTAL STATUS: Alert and oriented x3. Normal mood and affect.

LABORATORY/DIAGNOSTIC DATA: Sodium 140, potassium 3.8, chloride 110, CO_2 27, BUN 12, creatinine 0.7, glucose 83. Hemoglobin 9.3, hematocrit 28.4%, platelets 303,000, WBCs 6900. Troponin 0.01, CK 216. UTI screen positive.

IMPRESSION:
1. Chest pain.
2. Accelerated hypertension.
3. Gastroesophageal reflux disease.
4. History of iron deficiency anemia secondary to menorrhagia.
5. Urinary frequency.
6. Rule out urinary tract infection.
7. Medication noncompliance.

Proofreading & Editing Exercise

ABDOMINAL AORTOGRAM WITH LOWER EXTREMITY RUNOFF

CARDIAC IMAGING

PROCEDURE PERFORMED: Abdominal aortogram with lower extremity runoff.

CLINICAL HISTORY: The patient is a 66-year-old female with a history of intermittent claudication, as well as a family history of aneurysms. She comes in today for evaluation.

DESCRIPTION: The patient was brought to the catheterization laboratory in a stable, fasting condition. The right groin was prepped and draped in the usual fashion. A 5 French sheath was placed without difficulty in the left femoral artery using modified Seldinger technique. A 5 French marker pigtail catheter was placed in the abdominal aorta. Abdominal aortography was performed with the catheter just above the renal artery takeoff. The catheter was then brought down just above the aortoiliac junction, and digitally subtracted lower extremity angiography was performed bilaterally. Sheath was sewn in to be removed later in the postcatheterization area, after the catheter was removed over a wire. The patient tolerated the procedure without any problems in the laboratory. Contrast, total of 80 cc, was used.

FINDINGS:

ABDOMINAL AORTOGRAM: Smooth and free of significant disease.

LOWER EXTREMITIES RUNOFF:

Right lower extremity: The vessels were all seen pretty well and appeared to be free of significant plaque or ectasia.

Left lower extremity: The vessels of the left leg showed some minimal plaquing with maximal stenosis of 40% seen in the proximal common femoral artery.

IMPRESSION:

Pretty normal study. No evidence of significant occlusive disease.

RECOMMENDATIONS:

Reassurance.

Proofreading & Editing Exercise

Report #6

M-MODE, TWO-DIMENSIONAL AND DOPPLER ECHOCARDIOGRAM

CARDIOLOGY PROCEDURE REPORT

PROCEDURE: Echocardiogram.

REFERRING PHYSICIAN: XXXX

CLINICAL INDICATIONS: Syncope.

TYPE OF PROCEDURE: M-mode, 2-D and Doppler echocardiogram.

DESCRIPTION:

M-MODE AND TWO-DIMENSIONAL FINDINGS: Technically fair study done in standard, multiple views. Grossly, all four cardiac chambers have normal dimensions. The left ventricular systolic function is normal. Regional wall motion abnormalities are not detracted. Mild concentric left ventricular hypertrophy is noted; left ventricular ejection fraction is approximately 6%. Mitral, tricuspid and aortic valves appear to be grossly normal except for minimal calcification. Right-sided chambers are normal. Pericardial effusion is absent. No thrombi is seen in the left ventricle.

DOPPLER REPORT: Doppler echocardiographic analysis reveals trace mitral, tricuspid and aortic regurgitation. There is evidence of repaired relaxation of the left ventricle, consistent with diastolic dysfunction.

CONCLUSION:
1. Left ventricular systolic function is normal with an ejection fraction estimated to be approximately 6%.
2. Regional wall motion abnormalities are absent.
3. No significant valvular abnormalities are present.
4. Pericardial effusion is absent.
5. Intracardiac mass or thrombus is absent.

Proofreading & Editing Exercise

Report #7

HOLTER MONITOR

HOLTER MONITOR REPORT

PROCEDURE TYPE: A 24-hour Holter monitor.

INDICATIONS: A 74-year-old female complaining of "heart fluttering." Test is being done to evaluate.

FINDINGS:
1. Basic rhythm is sinus rhythm.
2. Average heart rate of 72 beats per minute, minimum heart rate 54 beats per minute, maximum heart rate 98 beats per minute at peak.
3. Competent PR interval, QRS, ST within normal limits.
4. Rare ventricular ectopic beats were seen; total number of ventricular ectopic beats in 24 hours were 6. There were no couplets, triplets, or runs of nonsustained or sustained ventricular tachycardia.
5. Rare atrial ectopic beats were seen; total number of atrial ectopic beats in 24 hours were 7. There were no runs of ventricular tachycardia.
6. No significant bradyarrhythmias seen.
7. Patient did not report any symptoms in the diary.

CONCLUSION:
1. Basic rhythm is sinus.
2. Rare atrial ectopic beats without runs of atrial tachycardia.
3. Rare ventricular ectopic beats without couplets, triplets, or runs of nonsustained or sustained ventricular tachycardia.
4. Patient did not report any symptoms in the diary.

Proofreading & Editing Exercise

THORACIC ARCH ARTERIOGRAPHY TO VISUALIZE CAROTID ARTERIES

VASCULAR IMAGING

PROCEDURES:

1. Thoracic arch arteriography.
2. Selective carotid arteriography.

PREPROCEDURE DIAGNOSIS:

Right carotid artery stenosis.

POSTPROCEDURE DIAGNOSIS:

Right carotid artery stenosis.

SUMMARY OF RADIOGRAPHIC FINDINGS:

Right carotid stenosis, 80%. Patent anterior and middle cerebral arteries. No intracoronary pathology. Easily cannulated common carotid artery with a Simmons 2.

INDICATIONS: This is a 71-year-old gentleman with renal insufficiency, COPD, coronary artery disease, CABG surgeries in 1983 and 1984, PTCA, CVA, and pacemaker, with episodic weakly stable angina and chest pain. He has an asymptomatic carotid artery stenosis.

TECHNIQUE:

After informed written consent was obtained, the patient was taken to the catheterization laboratory, placed in the supine position. After intravenous sedation was administered, the patient was prepped and draped in the usual sterile fashion. Via modified Seldinger technique, a direct puncture was made into the left common carotid artery. Wires and catheters were inserted to the level of the thoracic arch. A 5-French sheath was inserted with a pigtail catheter. Aortography was performed. A Simmons 2 catheter was used to cannulate the carotid arteries, and carotid angiography was performed. Upon termination of the procedure, all wires and catheters were removed. Patient tolerated the procedure well. The patient was sent to the recovery area in good condition.

FINDINGS:

The right internal carotid artery shows a carotid artery stenosis of approximately 80% to 90%, with involvement of the bifurcation; that is, it is not above or below the bifurcation. This is a very straight internal carotid artery. There is a normal arch configuration. All intracerebral vessels are observed. There is no intracerebral pathology.

FINAL IMPRESSION:

Right coronary artery stenosis, 80%.

Proofreading & Editing Exercise

HISTORY AND PHYSICAL EXAMINATION FOR SHORTNESS OF BREATH

HISTORY AND PHYSICAL EXAMINATION

CHIEF COMPLAINT/HISTORY OF PRESENT ILLNESS: Patient is a 78-year-old male who came to the emergency room this morning with shortness of breath. He stated that this started about two days ago when he had sharp, crampy pains across the lower chest that were quite severe. The next night, that is last night, he was severely short of breath, but it gradually started subsiding. The pains did not recur. This morning he awoke and again had severe shortness of breath, thus came to the emergency room for evaluation. No more chest pains have been reported. He describes no leg pain, however, there has been some slight swelling in the legs, particularly the left leg. He does have some mild, chronic leg cramping and swelling.

PAST MEDICAL HISTORY: Pertinent for a ventricular septal defect with secondary pulmonary hypertension. He also has hypertensive cardiovascular disease. The patient is obese. He also has a history of a nonischemic cardiomyopathy, probably related to the VSD, as well as a history of renal insufficiency, hyperlipidemia and AR.

PAST SURGICAL HISTORY: Previous surgeries as per old records.

ALLERGIES: NO KNOWN ALLERGIES TO MEDICATIONS.

MEDICATIONS: Routine medications currently include Singular 10 mg daily, Pravachol 20 mg daily, Toprol XL 50 mg daily, fosinopril 40 mg daily, Norvasc 5 mg daily, Plavix 7.5 mg daily, Clarinex 5 mg daily, spironolactone 25 mg daily, Lasix 40 mg daily.

SOCIAL HISTORY: Nonsmoker, nondrinker.

FAMILY HISTORY: Noncontributory.

REVIEW OF SYSTEMS: Essentially as above. Denies fevers or chills. Denies head or chest cold symptoms. Denies any worsening of his allergies or baseline breathing problems, except for above. No stomach pains or cramps, nausea or vomiting. Bowels have been moving regularly. No visible blood in the stool or urine. No burning or pain on urination.

PHYSICAL EXAMINATION:

GENERAL: Obese white male in no acute distress.

VITAL SIGNS: Vital signs in the emergency room included a blood pressure of 143/89, respirations 20, pulse 130 and regular, temperature 98.4, O2 saturation 95% on room air.

HEENT: EOMs full. Pupils reactive. Mucus membranes minimally dry.

(continued)

NECK: Supple, no adenopathy, no thyromegaly, no appreciable bruits in the neck.

CHEST: No adenopathy.

LUNGS: Lung fields revealed bibasilar crackles, more so on the left.

HEART: Regular; a harsh systolic murmur at the left upper sternal border. PMI was displaced bilaterally.

ABDOMEN: Soft, bowel sounds were active. No organomegaly. No masses, guarding or rebound.

RECTAL: Rectal referred to office.

EXTREMITIES: Full range of motion. Lower extremities had 2+ pedal edema, left greater than right, with bilateral venous stasis changes.

NEUROLOGIC: Grossly intact, without focal deficits.

DATA: Laboratory data include initial negative cardiac enzymes. D-dimer was 6.6. BMP was 562. Initial chemistries with a creatinine of 1.9, potassium 4.5, LFTs unremarkable, CBC was unremarkable, including a normal white cell count. A CT scan of the chest was reported, unofficially, as showing changes at both bases, consistent with pulmonary emboli.

IMPRESSION:
1. Probable bilateral basilar pulmonary emboli.
2. Shortness of breath, suspect secondary to above, however, cannot exclude acute decompensated heart failure.
3. History of ventricular septal defect with secondary pulmonary hypertension.
4. Nonischemic cardiomyopathy with prior history of congestive heart failure.
5. Obesity.
6. Renal insufficiency.
7. Hypertensive cardiovascular disease.
8. Hyperlipidemia.
9. Aortic regurgitation.

PLAN: At this time, patient will be admitted for further evaluation and therapy. He will be started immediately on heparin. Cardiology and pulmonary will be consulted. He will be kept on bed rest. Will continue his usual medications except for the Plavix. Monitor hemoglobin.
Patient may eventually require a Greenfield filter. Further treatment depends upon clinical course and findings.

Proofreading & Editing Exercise

Report #10

INFERIOR VENA CAVA FILTER PLACEMENT FOR PATIENT CONTRAINDICATED FOR ANTICOAGULATION

VASCULAR INTERVENTION PROCEDURE

PROCEDURE PERFORMED: Inferior vena cava filter placement.

PREPROCEDURE DIAGNOSIS: Pulmonary embolism.

POSTPROCEDURE DIAGNOSIS: Pulmonary embolism.

SURGEON: XXXX

INDICATIONS: Pulmonary embolism with DVT and bleeding; contraindication to anticoagulation.

ESTIMATED BLOOD LOSS: Minimal. No blood products given.

COUNTS: All counts were correct.

ACCESS: Right internal jugular vein.

SYSTEM: Trapeze.

PROCEDURE: After informed written consent was obtained, the patient was taken to the OR and placed in supine position. Intravenous sedation was administered. The patient was prepped and draped in the usual sterile fashion. After an appropriate amount of local anesthesia was given over the right internal jugular vein, a direct puncture was made into the vessel, and wires and catheters were inserted up into the inferior vena cava. An inferior venacavagram was performed and IVC filter was put below the renal veins. The patient tolerated the procedure well. There were no complications.

SUMMARY OF RADIOGRAPHIC FINDINGS:
1. Patient IVC.
2. Normal deployment of an inferior vena cava filter.

DISPOSITION: An IVC filter was placed just below the renal veins, in good position. There were no complications.

Proofreading & Editing Exercise

HISTORY AND PHYSICAL EXAMINATION FOR ATRIAL FIBRILLATION

HISTORY AND PHYSICAL EXAMINATION

CHIEF COMPLAINT: Chest pressure, palpitations.

HISTORY OF PRESENT ILLNESS: Patient is a 72-year-old white male with a past medical history significant for hypertension, coronary artery disease; he had a CABG done in March 2005. He had atrial fibrillation just prior to this surgery. He was doing very well until this morning, when he started having the feeling of palpations, plus feeling pressure in his chest, on the left side. He came into the emergency room for further evaluation. At home, he checked his blood pressure which was in the 90s. His heart rate went from the low 40s to as high as 150. In the emergency room, he had an initial evaluation with blood work and cardiac enzymes. She is being admitted to rule out MI protocol and evaluation of his atrial fibrillation.

PAST MEDICAL HISTORY: Significant for coronary artery disease, hypertension, and CABG in March 2005.

MEDICATIONS: At home he takes alprazolam, Zoloft, lisinopril, Plavix, Zocor, Toprol, Nexium, aspirin, and Allegra.

SOCIAL HISTORY: Patient lives at home with his wife. Patient does not smoke or drink alcohol.

FAMILY HISTORY: Noncontributory.

REVIEW OF SYSTEMS: Patient denies any temperature, any chills, any headache, any visual changes. Denies any shortness of breath, any cough. Denies any abdominal pain or any problem with bowels or bladder.

PHYSICAL EXAMINATION:

GENERAL: Physical exam shows a pleasant white man.

VITAL SIGNS: Blood pressure 112/48, heart rate 62, temperature 98.2.

HEENT: Head: Normocephalic, atraumatic. Eyes: Pupils round, reactive to light and accommodation; extraocular muscles intact. Mouth: Moist, no lesion.

NECK: No JVD, no bruit.

LUNGS: Clear to auscultation and percussion.

HEART: Regularly irregular. S1, S2. No murmur.

ABDOMEN: Soft; positive bowel sounds.

(continued)

EXTREMITIES: No edema.

NEUROLOGIC: Patient is alert, oriented, without any focal deficit.

LABORATORY/DIAGNOSTIC DATA: His labs show sodium 137, potassium 4.1, BUN 12, creatinine 0.9. White blood count 7500, hemoglobin and hematocrit of 42.6 and 14.7. His CPK initially was 39, troponin less than 0.01. ECG did not show any acute changes. A chest x-ray was within normal limits.

IMPRESSION:
1. Chest pressure, atrial fibrillation, new onset.
2. Hypertension.
3. History of coronary artery disease.

PLAN: Will admit patient to a monitored bed for rule out MI protocol and for rhythm evaluation. Will consult his cardiologist and will continue his home medications.

Proofreading & Editing Exercise

NORMAL PERSANTINE THALLIUM STRESS TEST

CARDIAC IMAGING

PROCEDURE: Persantine thallium

INDICATIONS: A 70-year-old admitted with atypical chest pain.

BASELINE: Resting electrocardiogram shows sinus rhythm, normal EKG.

PERSANTINE THALLIUM: The patient received an injection of Persantine per standard protocol. The resting heart rate was 70, which decreased to 82 after dipyridamole. The resting blood pressure was 104/50, which did not change. The patient denied chest pain. No ECG changes. No arrhythmias.

CONCLUSION:
1. Normal electrocardiographic response to dipyridamole.
2. Normal hemodynamic response to dipyridamole.
3. No chest pain during the test.
4. No arrhythmias.
5. The results of the thallium portion of the test were pending at the time of the dictation.

Proofreading & Editing Exercise

CONSULTATION FOR CHEST PAIN

CONSULTATION

ATTENDING: XXXX

CONSULTANT: XXXX

CHIEF COMPLAINT: Chest pain.

FINDINGS AND RECOMMENDATIONS OF CONSULTANT: The patient is a pleasant 84-year-old gentleman with multiple medical problems. He has a history of multivessel stenting, history of EF of 45% to 50%, with a recent admission for CHF, with elevated BNP, and also a urinary tract infection. According to his son, he was being transported in a van to a nursing home after a visit outside the nursing home and, in the process of transport, the patient developed chest pain. It may be musculoskeletal in nature, but the patient describes some heaviness associated with palpitations. He does have a history of coronary disease and has numerous other medical problems as well. He is a fairly poor historian, and most of the information obtained is form the patient's son. In terms of the ECG, he has evidence of T wave inversions seen in I and aVL. His first set of enzymes are pending. The patient also has severe peripheral vascular disease, has a history of chronic constipation, has a history of renal insufficiency, multiple myeloma as well and has had a history of a left lower extremity DVT leading to being placed on chronic anticoagulation. He also has a history of anemia and has had prior GI workup, the records of which are unavailable at this time. Patient describes some reproducible chest pain with palpation, but no diaphoresis and no radiation of the pain to the back; no orthopnea or PND.

REVIEW OF SYSTEMS: General: No fevers, chills, weight loss or weakness. Cardiovascular: See the HPI. Respiratory: See the HPI. GI: No nausea, vomiting, diarrhea; no abdominal pain or GI pain. Neurologic: No headaches, loss of consciousness, seizures, focal symptoms. Musculoskeletal: No joint swelling, neck pain, back pain. Eyes: No visual changes, painful discharge. ENT: No sore throat, earache, hearing changes. Hematologic: No anemia, abnormal bleeding, nodes, transfusion. Dermatologic: No rash, pruritus, lacerations, contusions. Psychiatric: No depression, A/V hallucinations, suicidal or homicidal ideations. GU: No dysuria, urgency, frequency, hesitancy, nocturia or hematuria. Endocrine: No heat or cold intolerance, no thyroid trouble.

PAST MEDICAL HISTORY: Positive as noted in HPI.

PAST SURGICAL HISTORY: Negative exact as noted above.

SOCIAL HISTORY: Negative for cigarette or alcohol use.

FAMILY HISTORY: Positive for hypertension.

(continued)

MEDICATIONS: Current medications include thalidomide, lactulose, Restoril; Pepcid 20 mg p.o. b.i.d.; Lopressor 12.5 p.o. b.i.d.; Zocor 40 mg p.o. q.h.s.; Medrol 4 mg p.o. q.d.; Norvasc 10 mg a day. The patient is also on Flomax 0.4 mg p.o. q. day; Synthroid 0.025 mg; Imdur 30 mg p.o. q. day; Sinemet 25/100; Senokot; Coumadin 3 mg a day; Lasix 20 mg p.o. q. day.

PHYSICAL EXAMINATION: A well-developed, well-nourished male, alert and comfortable. Vital signs show a blood pressure of 108/88, pulse of 64 and respiratory rate 18, temperature 98.9. Head was normal shape, no trauma. Eyes: Pupils equal, reactive to light and accommodation. Extraocular motions were intact. ENT: Nondeformed nose, normal lips, teeth and gums. Tongue and palate were clear. External canals were seen. Oral mucosa was moist with no exudate. Neck was supple, nontender, no masses, no JVD, trachea was midline. Cardiovascular: Regular rate and rhythm, with no murmurs, rubs or gallops. No pedal edema. Pulses were equal throughout. Respiratory effort: Lungs were clear to auscultation with no use of accessory muscles, no retractions. Chest: There is some reproducibility of the chest pain. GI: Normal bowel sounds, no masses. GU: Deferred. Musculoskeletal: Three limbs were present, with full range of motion. Back: No spasms, no spinous tenderness. Neurologic: Cranial nerves II through XII were intact. Patient was alert, oriented x3, with normal mental status. No lymphadenopathy appreciated.

LABORATORY DATA: First troponin was 0.03; ECG was described above; creatinine 1.3. White count 4600.

IMPRESSION:
1. History of chest pain.
2. Shortness of breath.
3. Coronary artery disease with multiple stents, reports unavailable.
4. Hypertension.
5. Hyperlipidemia.
6. Multiple myeloma.
7. History of renal artery stent.
8. History of DVT.
9. History of chronic anticoagulation with Coumadin therapy.
10. Chronic renal insufficiency.
11. Dementia.
12. History of below-knee amputation.
13. Hypothyroidism.
14. Benign prostatic hypertrophy.

PLAN:
After a long discussion with the patient and his son, we will rule out the patient by serial enzymes and follow. In terms of the subtherapeutic INR, the patient would probably need adjustment in the Coumadin dose.

Proofreading & Editing Exercise

Report #14

NORMAL THALLIUM STRESS TEST

CARDIAC IMAGING

PROCEDURE

Thallium stress test.

INDICATIONS

This is a 51-year-old with chest pain.

Baseline ECG shows normal sinus rhythm.

Patient underwent a treadmill stress test according to the standard Bruce protocol, exercising for 9 minutes, achieving a maximum heart rate of 143 beats per minute, which is greater than 85% of the target heart rate.

SYMPTOMS

No chest pain reported, no ECG changes noted.

Maximum blood pressure attained 200/100, a slightly hypertensive response, which is probably related to deconditioning.

No arrhythmias were noted. The recovery phase was uneventful. Approximately one minute prior to termination of the study, and at peak exercise, the patient was injected with thallium chloride intravenously, subsequently underwent nuclear imaging.

CONCLUSION

1. No electrocardiographic changes noted.
2. Low probability.
3. Duke score of 9.
4. No chest pain reported.
5. No arrhythmias noted.
6. Thallium pending at the time of this dictation.

Proofreading & Editing Exercise

CARDIOTHORACIC SURGICAL CONSULTATION FOR EVALUATION OF SUITABILITY FOR BYPASS GRAFT SURGERY

CONSULTATION REPORT

ATTENDING: XXXX

CONSULTANT: XXXX

REASON FOR CONSULTATION: A 62-year-old male with known coronary artery disease, with increasing angina pectoris, for myocardial revascularization.

HISTORY: A 62-year-old male with known coronary artery disease presented with progressive angina pectoris. He has a history of an acute myocardial infarction in October 2003, and has undergone placement of PTCA and stents to the right and diagonal coronary arteries. He also has a history of ventricular tachycardia and has undergone AICD placement. He has been followed by nuclear stress tests and diagnostic catheterizations. He notes increasing frequency of substernal chest pain. His last episode was in September; while exercising, he developed substernal discomfort radiating to his left hand, associated with diaphoresis. His symptoms resolved with two nitroglycerin tablets. Nuclear stress test in October 10, 2005, was noted to be abnormal, by history. Results, unfortunately, are not in the chart. Diagnostic catheterization was performed today, revealing significant 3-vessel coronary artery disease and moderately severe left ventricular dysfunction, with overall ejection fraction in the 30% range. Because of this, we were asked to see him in consultation for surgical opinion.

PAST MEDICAL HISTORY: Pertinent for diabetes, Niaspan intolerance, history of cataracts, hypothyroidism, hypertension.

MEDICATIONS: NovoLog 70/30, 12 units q.a.m., 8 units q.p.m.; hydrochlorothiazide 25 mg. q. day; Synthroid 0.05 mg. q. Tuesday-Thursday-Saturday-Sunday, 0.075 mg. Monday-Wednesday-Friday; amiodarone 100 mg. h.s.; aspirin 81 mg. q. day; Coreg 12.5 mg. b.i.d.; Plavix 75 mg. q. day, which last dose was last night; digoxin 0.25 mg. h.s.; Vasotec 5 mg. b.i.d.; Inspra 25 mg. h.s.; Zocor 40 mg. h.s.; glipizide ER 10 mg. b.i.d.

ALLERGIES: Ibuprofen and Niaspan.

FAMILY HISTORY: Denies coronary artery disease.

SOCIAL HISTORY: Previous tobacco abuse.

REVIEW OF SYSTEMS: No weight loss, weight gain, fever, chills. No eye pain, double vision; he has a history of cataracts. No eye discharge. No tinnitus, vertigo, frequent sore throats. He reports chest pain, no palpitations, no AICD discharge recently. No

(continued)

lower extremity edema. No hemoptysis, wheezing, pneumonia, or GI bleeding, hepatitis, gallbladder disease. No polyuria, polydipsia, polyphagia. He is on Synthroid. He reports prolonged bleeding secondary to aspirin and Plavix; prior to medications, he had no bleeding disorders. No cellulitis, no skin cancers. No lymphadenopathy. No TIA, amaurosis, frequent headaches. No mood swings, suicide intent, depression. No joint pain, back pain, muscle pain.

PHYSICAL EXAMINATION: In general, he is an alert male, on bed rest, in no acute distress. Blood pressure on admission was 120/76, pulse 74, regular; respirations 18 and unlabored; no fever. HEENT: Normocephalic, atraumatic. No deformities to the facial or head. Mucous membranes are moist. No scleral jaundice. Neck supple, with no carotid bruits, no JVD, no thyroid enlargement, nodules or tenderness. No carotid bruits. Lungs had good excursion, no use of accessory muscles; clear to auscultation. Heart: PMI displaced laterally. No palpable thrill. Regular rate and rhythm without murmur. Abdomen soft, nontender. No epigastric bruit, no hepatosplenomegaly, no abdominal aortic aneurysm, no tenderness; bowel sounds present. Extremity examination notes some right femoral artery pressure dressing, left femoral is 4+ without bruit. Popliteals are 3+, pedals are 3+. No clubbing, cyanosis or edema. Good saphenous veins. Musculoskeletal: No scoliosis, joint effusions, muscle wasting. Lymphatics: No supraclavicular, axillary or femoral lymphadenopathy. Neurological examination grossly intact. Motor, sensory and cranial nerves are intact. Oriented x3, to time, personal and place. Affect normal. Skin: No obvious skin lesions, skin cancer, cellulitis. Breasts: No abnormal breast masses. GU: Normal male. No CVA tenderness.

LABORATORY DATA: Diagnostic catheterization as noted. WBC 8100, hematocrit 45%, platelet count 180,000. Potassium 4.4, creatinine 1, glucose 231, INR 1.1.

IMPRESSION:

1. Coronary artery disease with:
   - Angina pectoris.
   - History of inferior wall myocardial infarction.
   - Left ventricular dysfunction.
   - Positive nuclear stress test.
2. Diabetes.
3. Previous tobacco abuse.
4. Hypertension.
5. Plavix and aspirin use.
6. Nonsustained ventricular tachycardia, status post automatic implantable cardioverter defibrillator.

PLAN:

Coagulation panel to assess bleeding tendencies. Myocardial revascularization following results of that. Risks, benefits, options, indications and alternatives to surgery have been discussed in detail with patient, family and wife. Following careful discussion and understanding, he has elected to proceed with the operation.

Proofreading & Editing Exercise

CONSULTATION FOR PATIENT WITH PERICARDITIS

CONSULTATION

ATTENDING:

XXXX

CONSULTANT:

XXXX

FINDINGS AND RECOMMENDATIONS OF CONSULTANT:

IMPRESSION:

1. Pericarditis with electrocardiographic changes consistent with pericarditis and pleuritic chest pain; respiratory tract infection approximately a month ago.
2. Occasional tobacco use.
3. Positive family history for coronary artery disease.

PLAN/RECOMMENDATION:

Obtain serial cardiac enzymes and EEGs; 2-D echocardiography to evaluate left ventricular systolic function. If enzymes are negative, then proceed with treadmill stress testing.

The patient is a 33-year-old male who was in his usual state of health up until a week ago when he began developing chest discomfort with inspiration. However, on the morning of admission, he woke up with stabbing chest pain, worsened by inspiration, but not with moving or palpation. With the pain persisting, patient sought medical attention at the emergency room where he was evaluated and subsequently admitted. His pain went away with analgesics. Patient denies a history of coronary artery disease in the past, has never had cardiac testing. No congestive heart failure, valvular or rheumatic heart disease.

CARDIAC RISK FACTORS:

Occasional tobacco use, but no dyslipidemia, diabetes or hypertension.

FAMILY HISTORY:

Questionable. He states his father died of a myocardial infarction at the age of 30?

REVIEW OF SYSTEMS:

Significant for above. History of genital herpes. Denies CVA, seizure disorder, thyroid disease, asthma, bronchitis, emphysema, peptic ulcer disease or GI bleeding, viral hepatitis or pancreatitis, change in bowel habits, involuntary weight loss, kidney stones, renal insufficiency, gout, DVT, claudication, pulmonary embolism or malignancies.

(continued)

PAST SURGICAL HISTORY:

Status post appendectomy in childhood.

ALLERGIES:

No known drug allergies.

MEDICATIONS:

Prior to admission, Valtrex.

SOCIAL HISTORY:

No alcohol or drug abuse. He is a smoker, smoking a few cigarettes occasionally.

PHYSICAL EXAMINATION:

Physical examination reveals a well-developed, well-nourished male, in no apparent distress. Vital signs: Blood pressure is 130/70, pulse is 18 and regular, respiratory rate 80. HEENT atraumatic, normocephalic. Anicteric sclerae. Neck veins not distended at a 30-degree angle, carotid upstrokes not delayed, no bruits. Lungs are clear to auscultation and percussion. PMI is not displaced, first and second heart sounds are regular without gallops or murmurs. Abdomen is soft, nontender, with normoactive bowel sounds. No visceromegaly, masses or bruits. Extremities without edema, cyanosis or clubbing. Peripheral pulses are intact.

LABORATORY DATA:

Sodium 141, potassium 3.7, BUN 18, creatinine 0.9. Cardiac enzymes x2 negative for myocardial necrosis. WBC on admission was 12,100, but this morning 6,800; hemoglobin 14.7, hematocrit 42.3%, platelet count 279,000. D-dimer was normal at 0.7. Chest x-ray reported as normal, will review.

Proofreading & Editing Exercise

Report #17

ABNORMAL TRANSESOPHAGEAL ECHOCARDIOGRAM

ECHOCARDIOGRAM STUDY

PROCEDURE: Transesophageal echocardiogram.

INDICATIONS: A 73-year-old female with rheumatic heart disease, history of mitral valve prolapse, and recently documented echocardiogram suggesting possible ruptured chordae with moderate to severe mitral regurgitation reported.

LOCAL ANESTHETIC: Cetacaine spray 10%.

INTRAVENOUS SEDATION: Versed 4 mg and Demerol 50 mcg.

PROCEDURE DETAILS: Consent was obtained for a transesophageal echocardiogram study. The risks and the benefits of the procedure were explained to the patient in detail. The patient was placed in the left lateral decubitus position and after appropriate sedation and local anesthetic were given. While under constant heart rate, blood pressure and pulse oximetry monitoring, the OmniPlane transesophageal echocardiogram probe was inserted via the posterior pharynx into the esophagus, with multiple views obtained. Subsequently, the probe was removed without difficulty. The patient tolerated the procedure well, with no apparent complications.

FINDINGS: The left ventricle is normal in size, internal dimensions and wall thickness. The ventricle is only partially visualized in the TEE view, due to the heart beating off axis. Right ventricle is normal in size and function. The left and right atrium are mildly dilated. The interatrial septum is intact. Color flow study across the interatrial septum demonstrates no evidence of right-to-left or left-to-right shunting. Left atrial appendage is partially visualized and appears to be unremarkable. Mitral valve is structurally abnormal. The mitral valve anterior leaflet is thickened and myxomatous; it demonstrates prolapse. There are two separate jets of mitral regurgitation noted, demonstrating moderate mitral regurgitation. No stenosis is seen. There is no evidence for ruptured chordae. The aortic valve leaflets are visualized. They are grossly trileaflet; they are mildly thickened. The aortic valve leaflets open without stenosis and close without prolapse. Pulmonic and tricuspid valves appear unremarkable. There is evidence for mild tricuspid regurgitation. No pericardial effusion is seen. There is mild to moderate atherosclerotic plaquing of the thoracic aorta. The ascending and descending aorta appears essentially normal.

CONCLUSION:
1. Normal left ventricular size and systolic function.
2. Mitral valve prolapse with moderate mitral regurgitation. No evidence for ruptured chordae.
3. Mildly thickened aortic valve leaflets with associated mild aortic regurgitation.
4. Remaining valves are structurally unremarkable.
5. No thrombus or vegetation is identified.
6. No pericardial effusion is seen.
7. Mild to moderate atherosclerotic plaquing of the thoracic descending aorta is seen.

Proofreading & Editing Exercise

CONSULTATION FOR PATIENT WITH HEART MURMUR (PEDIATRIC)

CONSULTATION REPORT

REQUESTING: XXXX

CONSULTANT: XXXX

REASON FOR CONSULTATION: I was asked to evaluate this baby boy because of the finding of heart murmur.

This is a 2-day-old male newborn who was born by cesarean section delivery because of previous C-section. His Apgar scores were 8 at one minute and 9 at five minutes. He required oxygenation right after delivery because of mild respiratory distress that was thought to be transient tachypnea of the neonate. His birth weight was 3.178 kg. He is now asymptomatic from a cardiovascular standpoint. There is no history of pallor, cyanosis, easy fatigability or syncope. He is progressing nicely with p.o. enteral feedings. He is on ampicillin and gentamicin because of his respiratory distress soon after delivery. His blood cultures are negative at 48 hours. His CBC is normal. His chest x-ray is normal as well. Heart murmur was heard today on physical examination and thought to be compatible with a holosystolic murmur, likely a ventricular septal defect. Cardiac consultation was requested.

He is the third child of a 25-year-old mom. His older siblings are healthy. His family history is negative for congenital heart disease or sudden death.

Physical examination revealed a full-term newborn, active and alert, with a weight of 3035 gm. His temperature was 98.5, heart rate was 148 per minute, respiratory rat was 38 per minute and unlabored. His oxygen saturation was 96% on room air. His blood pressure was obtained in all four extremities. The right arm was 64/42, right leg 75/50, left arm 78/44, and left leg 78/42 mmHg. His mucous membranes were moist and pink. Bruits were not auscultated. His carotid pulses were strong and symmetric. JVD was not seen. His thyroid gland was not palpable. Adenopathies were not palpated. His lungs were clear to auscultation. Bilateral breath sounds were heard. His precordium was normally active on chest exam. The first and second heart sounds were both normal; a grade 3/6 holosystolic murmur was heard at the left sternal border, radiating over the precordium. Diastolic murmurs were not heard. Clicks were not heard. His abdomen was soft; his liver was 1 cm below the costal margin. Organomegaly was not palpated. Abdominal bruits were not heard. Normal male genitalia was noted. His peripheral pulses were strong and symmetric, without brachial-femoral delay noted. Peripheral edema was not seen.

An ECG demonstrated sinus rhythm with normal intervals for age. Right axis deviation with right ventricular prominence was noted; that is a normal finding for a neonate. A cardiac ultrasound was reviewed and interpreted by me. It demonstrated

(continued)

a patent foramen ovale and trivial left peripheral branch pulmonic stenosis, which are physiologic findings for age. Additionally, a small (2- to 3-mm) mid muscular ventricular septal defect with left-to-right shunt was noted. The aortic arch was normal. PDA was not seen.

SUMMARY:

In summary, this newborn's evaluation is consistent with a small ventricular septal defect of no hemodynamic significance at this point. My only recommendation is bacterial endocarditis prophylaxis when at risk for bacteremia, and a follow-up appointment in the outpatient cardiac clinic in approximately 3 months. The findings were communicated to his mother and the attending physician.

Thanks for this consultation.

Proofreading & Editing Exercise

TILT TABLE TEST

TILT TABLE STUDY

PROCEDURE
Tilt table study.

CLINICAL HISTORY
A very pleasant 88-year-old woman with recurrent syncope and recent myocardial infarction.

DESCRIPTION
The patient underwent tilt table testing on a tilt table with a foot board for weight bearing. Baseline heart rate and blood pressure determinations were made. After being in the upright position for roughly 10 minutes without symptoms or hemodynamic abnormalities, one spray of sublingual nitroglycerin was administered. During this time period, she had reproduction of clinical symptoms with near-syncope as well as sudden and profound drop in systolic blood pressure to 50 mmHg. No significant bradycardia was noted. The table was brought back down to horizontal. She tolerated the procedure quite well.

FINDINGS
1. No pathologic pauses with right-sided or left-sided coronary sinus massage.
2. Positive study for neurocardiogenic syncope with primary vasodepressor component with reproduction of symptoms.

RECOMMENDATIONS
Given these findings, I recommend reinstitution of surgical compression stockings. Will add Florinef 0.1 mg daily therapy. Will discuss these with her cardiologist.

Proofreading & Editing

STENTING OF LEFT ANTERIOR DESCENDING ARTERY

PERCUTANEOUS CORONARY INTERVENTION

PROCEDURE: Stenting of proximal left anterior descending with 3.5 x 8-mm Cypher drug-eluting stent. Stenting of mid left anterior descending with 3 x 18-mm Cypher drug-eluting stent. Intracoronary nitroglycerin for spasm.

CLINICAL HISTORY: Patient is a 69-year-old female with a history of coronary artery disease, for stenting of LAD.

DESCRIPTION: Consent was obtained after explaining the risks, benefits and alternatives, risks involving renal failure, retroperitoneal hemorrhage, bleeding, stroke and imponderables. A 7-French sheath was placed in the right femoral artery. An XB 3.5 guide was used to cannulate the left main. An IQ wire was placed in the distal LAD. Nitroglycerin 200 mcg was given to diffuse spasm. Angiomax was administered; patient was already on aspirin and Plavix.

This was followed by primary stenting of proximal LAD with a 3.5 x 8-mm Cypher drug-eluting stent which was employed to 14 atmospheres. Stenosis was reduced from 70% to 0%. The mid LAD was stented with a 3 x 18-mm Cypher drug-eluting stent which was employed to 18 atmospheres. Stenosis was reduced from 70% to 0%. No evidence of any dissection or embolization. Excellent results.

IMPRESSION: Successful stenting of proximal and mid left anterior descending artery with Cypher drug-eluting stents, with excellent results.

Proofreading & Editing Exercise   Report #21

LEFT HEART CATHETERIZATION AND VENTRICULOGRAPHY IN PATIENT WITH CARDIOMYOPATHY

OPERATIVE REPORT

PROCEDURE: Left heart catheterization, ventriculogram.

INDICATIONS: A 65-year-old admitted with chest pain, positive troponins, stress test showing ischemia.

DESCRIPTION: After informed consent was obtained, the patient was brought to the cardiac catheterization laboratory where the right groin was prepped and draped in the usual sterile fashion. Local anesthesia was achieved using 1% lidocaine. Seldinger technique was used to cannulate the right femoral artery. We used a 5-French system, JL4, JR4, angled pigtail for single-plane ventriculogram. The patient tolerated the procedure without complications.

HEMODYNAMIC FINDINGS: The aortic pressure was 135/77. The LV was 135 with an end-diastolic of 14. There was no gradient on pullback across the aortic valve.

ANGIOGRAPHIC FINDINGS:

LEFT MAIN CORONARY ARTERY: The left main was free of significant disease.

CIRCUMFLEX: The circumflex was a moderate-sized vessel giving off two marginal branches. The did not appear to be significant disease involving these vessels.

LEFT ANTERIOR DESCENDING: The LAD was a moderate-sized vessel giving off three diagonal branches. The first diagonal was moderate in size; second and third were quite small. There did not appear to be any evidence of significant disease involving the LAD or diagonal system.

RIGHT CORONARY ARTERY: The right coronary artery was a moderate-sized vessel, giving off a PDA and a PL branch, both with minimal irregularity. The distal PDA and PL branch are small, but no significant vocal stenosis was appreciated.

VENTRICULOGRAM: Single plane ventriculogram showed the ejection fraction was significantly impaired at about 35%.

CONCLUSION:
1. Minimal coronary artery disease.
2. Elevated left ventricular end-diastolic pressure.
3. Moderate left ventricular dysfunction, ejection fraction 35%.

RECOMMENDATIONS: This patient appears to have a nonischemic cardiomyopathy. The interesting fact is that her daughter also has cardiomyopathy and required defibrillator placement. Hopefully her ventricle will stabilize with ACE-inhibitor and beta-blocker therapy.

Proofreading & Editing Exercise

DOBUTAMINE STRESS ECHOCARDIOGRAM

CARDIAC IMAGING

PROCEDURE: Dobutamine stress echocardiogram.

INDICATION: The patient is a 34-year-old female with chest pain. The patient was unable to have a nuclear stress test due to a recent menstrual cycle and, therefore, a dobutamine stress echocardiogram was recommended.

PROTOCOL: After informed consent was obtained, the patient was infused with IV dobutamine starting at 5 mcg/kg/min, increased to a total of 30 mcg/kg/min. The patient was given 0.5 mg of IV atropine to achieve the peak heart rate needed. Her peak heart rate was approximately 160 beats per minute. Peak blood pressure was approximately 150/72. She did have some chest pain and shortness of breath during the protocol.

ELECTROCARDIOGRAPHIC EVALUATION: At baseline, the patient had an ECG which revealed a normal sinus rhythm, nonspecific ST-T wave changes in the inferolateral leads. During peak heart rate, the patient had less than 1 mm of horizontal ST-segment depression. There were no malignant atrial or ventricular arrhythmias noted.

ECHOCARDIOGRAPHIC EVALUATION: Two-dimensional and Doppler ultrasonography were performed in the usual manner. At baseline, the patient had grossly normal left ventricular size and wall thickness with left ventricular ejection fraction estimated at approximately 60%. No significant wall motion abnormalities are noted. There was no significant valvular regurgitation noted. The cardiac valves appear to be structurally within normal limits. Optison was used for the apical views. At peak heart rate, the patient had appropriate augmentation of left ventricular systolic function. No significant wall motion abnormalities are noted. There was appropriate decrease in left ventricular size.

IMPRESSION:
1. No electrocardiographic evidence for ischemia noted.
2. Echocardiographic evaluation reveals no significant wall motion abnormalities. There is an appropriate decrease in left ventricular size.

Proofreading & Editing Exercise

Report #23

ECHOCARDIOGRAM WITH DOPPLER

DOPPLER STUDY

PROCEDURE: Echocardiogram with Doppler.

CLINICAL HISTORY: A 75-year-old man with acute anterior wall myocardial infarction. This study is to evaluate LV function, presence of apical clot, and complications of myocardial infarction.

Procedure of two-dimensional echocardiography, M-mode, and complete Doppler was performed. The quality of the study is good.

FINDINGS:

M-MODE: Left ventricular end-diastolic dimension 3.6 cm, end-systolic dimension 2.7 cm. Interventricular septal thickness 1.7 cm, posterior wall 1.5 cm. Ejection fraction estimated at 45% to 50%. Left atrial size 3.8 cm. Aortic root 3.2 cm.

TWO-DIMENSIONAL: There is a moderate size anteroapical wall motion abnormality. This is moderately to severely hypokinetic, clearly not akinetic. There is no paradoxic motion of the septa. Remaining walls appear to move normally with preserved LV systolic function, ejection fraction around 50%. There is mild mitral annular calcification with mild sclerotic changes of the mitral and aortic valves. The aortic valve is clearly tricuspid, without stenosis. No pericardial effusion is seen. There are no other abnormal calcifications.

DOPPLER: Trace mitral regurgitation is seen, as well as mild tricuspid insufficiency. Pulmonary artery pressure is normal at 33 mmHg. The E-to-A ratio is abnormal, suggesting diastolic noncompliance.

IMPRESSION:
1. Mildly-reduced left ventricular systolic function, ejection fraction 50%, with anteroapical wall motion abnormality, consistent with patient's clinical history of anterior wall myocardial infarction.
2. Mild innocent changes of the mitral and aortic valves, with no hemodynamically significant flow abnormalities.
3. Normal pulmonary pressures.
4. The E-to-A ratio is abnormal, suggesting diastolic noncompliance, which is typical for an infarcted ventricle.
5. No apical clot is identified.

Proofreading & Editing Exercise

Report #24

PACEMAKER INSERTION (PEDIATRIC)

PACEMAKER REPORT

PREOPERATIVE DIAGNOSIS:
1. Status post repair of pulmonary atresia and tetralogy of Fallot.
2. Third-degree heart block.

POSTOPERATIVE DIAGNOSIS:
1. Status post repair of pulmonary atresia and tetralogy of Fallot.
2. Third-degree heart block.

OPERATION:
Pacemaker insertion, ventricular pacing, ventricular sensing, inhibited mode, epicardial, subrectus.

SURGEON:
XXXX

ANESTHESIA:
Given by pediatric intensivist.

INDICATIONS:
This 2-week-old girl was born with complex pulmonary atresia and tetralogy of Fallot, and underwent complete repair as a neonate. Postoperatively, the baby manifested sustained third-degree atrioventricular block and was pacing using the temporary leads placed intraoperatively. With absence of return of conduction after 1-1/2 weeks, a pacemaker is now justified.

PROCEDURE:
Following induction of anesthesia, the baby was sterilely prepped and draped and given IV antibiotics. A midline subxiphoid vertical incision was made and carried down into the left rectus sheath. The rectus muscle was reflected anteriorly and a plane developed between the posterior rectus sheath and rectus muscle to develop a generator packet. The incision was extended to the xiphoid process, then dissection carried out to the diaphragmatic edge and into the pericardial cavity; the inferior wall of the right ventricle was exposed. A steroid-eluding, single 15-cm long epicardial lead was then fixated to the inferior wall of the right ventricle using two 5-0 Prolene mattress stitches. The lead was tested and had an R wave amplitude of 8.2 mV, with a pacing threshold of 0.9 V and an impedance of 439 ohms. The wound was thoroughly irrigated with antibiotic-saline solution. The lead was then connected to a Medtronic Enpulse SR single-chamber generator, model #E2SR01, and the generator was placed in the pocket. After further antibiotic irritation, the temporary pacing leads were removed, given that there was good pacing using the generator. The wound was then closed in layers with running absorbable suture. In particular, the

(continued)

rectus sheath was reapproximated to the contralateral side very carefully to avoid epicardial hernia. Monofilament nylon was used to close the skin, and then a dry dressing was placed.

The baby tolerated the procedure apparently well. Care was continued after taking the baby back to the cardiac intensive care unit.

Proofreading & Editing Exercise

TRANSCATHETER OCCLUSION OF PATENT FORAMEN OVALE

PERCUTANEOUS CORONARY INTERVENTION

PROCEDURE: Transcatheter occlusion of patent foramen ovale

PREPROCEDURE DIAGNOSIS: Patent foramen ovale

POSTPROCEDURE DIAGNOSIS: Patent foramen ovale

INDICATIONS: This 64-year-old lady presented with a stroke ten days ago. This was confirmed to be an embolic event, with no other source identified. She was felt to be a poor candidate for anticoagulation therapy, and after discussion with her cardiologist and neurologist, we agreed to consider transcatheter occlusion of a patent foramen ovale. Detailed discussion was undertaken with patient and her hubby prior to embarking on the procedure, including the risks, benefits and alternatives to the use of device occlusion of the patent foramen ovale. Informed consent was obtained.

PROCEDURE DETAILS: Patient was sedated with Versed and fentanyl, as supervised by cardiac anesthesia. Xylocaine 2% local anesthesia was infiltrated into the right groin, after prepping and draping in the usual manner. Percutaneous entry into the right femoral vein was obtained and a 10-French sheath inserted. This allowed passage of a multipurpose catheter across the patent foramen ovale. Utilizing the multipurpose catheter, a 0.035-inch Amplatz wire was introduced from the right atrium to the left atrium, across the patent foramen ovale, and anchored in the left lower pulmonary vein. A 3-cm balloon seizing catheter was introduced across the patent foramen ovale. By fluoroscopy, the patent foramen ovale balloon sized to 9 mm.

It should be noted that the patient was a poor candidate for general anesthesia, in view of the decreased ejection fraction; hence, she was not subjected to transesophageal echocardiography.

Utilizing fluoroscopy as a Marker, the short 10-French sheath was exchanged for a long 10-French sheath. An occlusion device was prepared in the usual manner and introduced via the 10-French sheath to the atrium. The distal left atrial portion of the device was delivered and, by fluoroscopy, confirmed to be against the left atrial side of the septum. Following this, the right atrial portion of the device was released as well. By fluoroscopy, the device was seen to be in excellent position. The device was released without complication. The 10-French sheath was exchanged for a short 10-French sheath, in order to allow for VasoSeal-assisted hemostasis. Catheters were removed, bleeding stopped by local pressure.

(continued)

Patient was conscious and talking throughout the procedure and experienced no discomfort. The patient was transferred back to her floor for subsequent recovery.

Following the procedure, the patient will be maintained on aspirin 325 mg and Plavix 75 mg daily for a period of 6 months. Patient will have a chest x-ray as well as an echocardiogram 24 hours following the procedure and be maintained on 3 doses of Ancef over 24 hours.

Proofreading & Editing Exercise

ELECTROPHYSIOLOGIC STUDY

ELECTROPHYSIOLOGIC STUDY

PROCEDURE: Electrophysiologic study.

CLINICAL HISTORY: A very pleasant 75-year-old gentleman with ischemic heart disease, with syncopal episode associated with motor vehicle accident and severe trauma. Patient has undergone recent PCI. He is aware of the risks, benefits, and alternatives to proceeding with electrophysiologic study for further assessment.

He Is aware that these risks include, but are not limited to, infection, death, stroke, myocardial infarction, vessel damage, limb damage, pain, pneumothorax, deep venous thrombosis, pulmonary embolus, need for vascular repair, need for transfusion, need for device and/or lead repoisoning, and the possibility that this might not improve, and even worsen, his situation. He understands and wishes to proceed with electrophysiologic study.

PROCEDURE/TECHNIQUE: After informed consent was obtained, the patient was brought to the EP laboratory in a fasting state. He was prepped and draped in the usual sterile fashion with multiple layers of Betadine. Pilocaine 1% infiltration was used to achieve local anesthesia over the left inguinal area. Using a #18-gauge needle and a 0.035 guidewire, access was obtained into the left femoral vein. Over the guidewire, a 5-French sheath was advanced into this vessel. Using identical technique at 2 separate sites along the course of the left femoral vein, two 6-French sheaths were advanced. Through these sheaths, one 6-French and two 5-French, 5-mm quadripolar electrode catheters were advanced, using fluoroscopic and electrocardiographic guidance, to positions in the high right atrium, right ventricular apex, and to a position across the tricuspid annulus such that a Hiss bundle electrogram could be carefully mapped and recorded. After baseline intervals and pacing thresholds were obtained, RA and RV incremental pacing and programmed stimulation were performed. Sinus node recovery times were performed. Carotid sinus massage was performed. At the end of the procedure, all catheters and sheaths were removed. He tolerated the procedure quite well and returned to the recovery area in stable condition.

FINDINGS:
1. At baseline, intracardiac intervals are normal, with an A-H interval of 90 msec and an H-V interval of 52 msec.
2. Markedly abnormal sinus node function is demonstrated. Corrected sinus node recovery times are reproducibly increased up to 3500 msec. This is a reproducible finding.
3. AV nodal function is normal with an antegrade AV nodal refractory period of 700/440 and an antegrade Wenckebach cycle length of 450 msec.
4. No supraventricular arrhythmias are inducible.

(continued)

5. There is no evidence of an accessory bypass track. All conductions are central through the AV node in both the antegrade and retrograde directions; both antegrade and retrograde Wenckebach are seen.

6. No pathologic pauses or hypotension is noted with right-sided or left-sided carotid sinus massage.

7. Episodes of ventricular tachycardia are reproducibly inducible during drive cycle lengths of 400 msec, from both the right ventricular apex and the right ventricular outflow tract. These episodes are prolonged but self terminating.

CONCLUSION: This is a markedly abnormal electrophysiologic study with both ventricular tachycardia and evidence for sinus node dysfunction. Given the patient's ischemic myopathy, syncope with trauma, I will recommend a dual-chamber transvenous pectoral defibrillator.

Proofreading & Editing Exercise

Report #27

ATRIOVENTRICULAR CANAL REPAIR WITH LIGATION OF PATENT DUCTUS ARTERIOSUS (PEDIATRIC)

OPERATIVE REPORT

PREOPERATIVE DIAGNOSES
1. Atrioventricular canal defect, transitional.
2. Ductus arteriosus.
3. Down syndrome.

POSTOPERATIVE DIAGNOSES
1. Atrioventricular canal defect, transitional.
2. Ductus arteriosus.
3. Down syndrome.

OPERATION
1. Atrioventricular canal defect repair, on cardiopulmonary bypass.
2. Ligation of ductus arteriosus.

SURGEON
XXXX

ASSISTANT
XXXX

ANESTHESIA
General.

INDICATIONS
This 7-month-old, 6-kg child with Down syndrome has a transitional atrioventricular canal defect. The child has been growing well, without overt failure. A recent follow-up echocardiogram revealed an atrioventricular canal defect with only a very small ventricular component to the shunt, with the septal crest largely covered over by accessory valve leaflet tissue. There was a moderate primum component to the canal, and a small patent foramen ovale. There was a cleft in the left atrioventricular valve, with minimal regurgitation.

PROCEDURE
Following induction of anesthesia, the baby was sterilely prepped and draped and given IV antibiotics. A midline chest incision was made, carried down through the sternum with a saw, and a retractor placed. The thymus gland was excised and the pericardium was cleaned off, a patch excised and tanned in glutaraldehyde, and the remaining pericardium suspended on sutures. The ascending aorta and superior vena cava were resected out. The ductus arteriosus was exposed and ligated with a 2-0 Tevdek tie. Heparin 300 units/kg was given, bicaval cannulation completed, and cardiopulmonary begun with cooling to 28 degrees. Tourniquets were placed around

(continued)

the cavae, a vent was placed through the right superior pulmonary vein into the left ventricle, and a cardioplegic catheter placed. The aorta was occluded, and 25 cc/kg of crystalloid cardioplegia given, with maintenance doses of 10 cc/kg given every 20 to 30 minutes. The caval tourniquets were then tightened, an oblique right atriotomy made, and the edges suspended on traction stitches. The ventricles were suctioned of blood, then the canal defect was inspected. The primam defect was moderate, at most. We could not appreciate a ventricular component by direct but gentle probing. There was abundant attachments to the crest of the septum. Saline distention revealed a rather linear cleft between the superior and inferior bridging leaflets of the left AV valve, and a well-developed posterior leaflet. Though we could visualize the cleft through the primam defect, we could not readily expose it for closure. Therefore, we enlarged the primam defect by excising a small amount of septum from the superior lateral border of the defect. The left AV valve could now be much better visualized. The first marginal chords were located on the superior and inferior bridging leaflets, near the coaptation with the posterior leaflet. A 7-0 Prolene suture was then taken through the superior and inferior leaflets at this location and tied with three knots. One end was tagged, and this served to bring the valve up through the primam defect, where the cleft was now easily visualized. The cleft was then closed, running each arm of the 7-0 Prolene suture up to the septum. The cleft was not complete all the way to the septum, so we ran it to the sturdy accessory valve tissue at the base, near the septal attachments. The valve was then tested with saline distention and was completely competent, and had an adequate orifice. The small ventricular level shunt, if any, was probably at the location of the cleft near the crest of the septum. We closed this area with a pledgetted mattress suture of 6-0 Ethibond, and then tied this stitch to the Prolene cleft-closure stitch. The primam defect was then closed with the tanned pericardial patch and running 6-0 Prolene suture, with care taken to avoid the conduction system, as best as possible. The left atrium was distended with saline and the lungs ventilated to evacuate air prior to completion of this closure.

Rewarming was started. The patent foramen ovale was closed with a single mattress stitch of 6-0 Prolene. The right atrium was closed with doubly run 6-0 Prolene. After standard de-airing maneuvers, including an ascending aortic vent, the aortic clamp was removed, and the heart was reprofused. It began beating in spontaneous sinus rhythm during warming. The caval tourniquets were removed. Two right atrial catheters were placed and secured to the skin. A right ventricular pacing wire was placed and secured with a ground wire. Dopamine 5 mcg/kg per minute was started. With good cardiac activity, and after appropriate warming to 37 degrees core temperature, cardiopulmonary bypass was discontinued. Transesophageal echocardiography revealed no residual atrial or ventricular level shunts, and only trivial left AV valve and right AV valve regurgitation. The cannulas were thus removed, and protamine sulfate given. Hemostasis was rendered. The mediastinum was irrigated with antibiotic saline solution. The 16-French drain tube was placed and secured to the skin. After a final inspection and confirmation of counts, the chest was closed in layers with interrupted sternal wires and layers of running absorbable suture. An On-Q catheter was placed continuous Marcaine infusion. A dry dressing was placed. The baby tolerated the procedure apparently well, and care was continued in the cardiac ICU.

Proofreading & Editing Exercise   Report #28

DUAL-CHAMBER AUTOMATIC IMPLANTABLE CARDIOVERTER DEFIBRILLATOR IMPLANTATION

CARDIOLOGY PROCEDURE REPORT

PROCEDURE: Dual-chamber defibrillator insertion.

INDICATIONS: Patient experiencing syncopal episodes, with significant conduction abnormalities as noted on a recent EP study. An AICD is expected to prevent these arrhythmias as well as prevent sudden cardiac death.

PROCEDURE/TECHNIQUE: After informed consent was obtained, the patient was brought to the electrophysiology laboratory. She was prepped and draped in surgical fashion. The right subclavian area was anesthetized with 1% Xylocaine. Using modified Seldinger technique, the right subclavian vein was cannulated twice, and guide wires were advanced to the level of the inferior vena cava and secured with hemostats. An area 1 inch inferior was anesthetized with 1% Xylocaine. Using a #15 scalpel, the skin was incised, and the incision was carried down to the prepectoral fascia using Bovie cautery. The prepectoral fascia was then split using scissors, and dissection was carried out inferiorly to create a pocket and superiorly to incorporate both wires into the wound. The first guide wire was then used to advance an 11-French tear-away sheath under fluoroscopic guidance into the left subclavian vein. The sheath was in turn used to advance a Medtronic ventricular lead, model #5706, serial #XXXX. This lead was advanced under fluoroscopic guidance to the level of the inferior vena cava. The sheath was torn away and pressure held over the puncture site until hemostasis was obtained. This lead was then fitted with a curved stylet and advanced into the right ventricular outflow tract. Using a straight stylet, the lead was slowly withdrawn until it advanced into the right ventricular apex. The active fixation helix was then deployed using the supplied tool. The lead was then tested and found to have R waves of 8.3 mV with a pacing threshold of 0.4 V at 0.5 msec pulse width and an impedance of 468 ohms. Ten-volt pacing did not elicit any diaphragmatic capture. These values were judged acceptable, so the lead was sutured into place with #0 silk and the supplied sleeve. The second guide wire was then used to advance a 7-French tear-away sheath under fluoroscopic guidance in the left subclavian vein. This sheath was in turn used to advance a Medtronic atrial lead, model #5706, serial #XXXX. This lead was advanced under fluoroscopic guidance to the level of the inferior vena cava. The sheath was torn away and pressure was held over the puncture site until hemostasis was obtained. The lead was then fitted with a J-shape stylet and advanced into the area of the right atrial appendage. With four clockwise turns of the lead body, the lead was actively fixed in place. The stylet was withdrawn, and the lead was tested and found to have P waves of 6.8 mV with a pacing threshold of 0.5 V at 1 msec pulse width and an impedance of 686 ohms. Ten-volt pacing did not elicit any

(continued)

phrenic nerve capture. These values were judged acceptable, so the lead was sutured in place with #0 silk and the supplied sleeve. The leads were then disconnected from the Pacing Systems Analyzer and connected to a Medtronic generator, model #4768, serial #XXXX. Each lead was identified by its markings and serial numbers and connected to the appropriate port, with the distal coil being connected to the high voltage negative pole. All connections were secured with a torque wrench. The device was then implanted into the newly created pocket, after a lavage with copious amounts of antibiotic-saline solution. The device was secured to the floor of the pocket using a #0 silk stitch. We then proceeded with device testing.

Through the device, P waves were 6 mV and R waves were 8 mV. Pacing thresholds were 0.5 V at 0.5 msec in both channels. Atrial impedance was 680 ohms and ventricular impedance was 490 ohms. The patient was then heavily sedated with fentanyl and Versed. Using T-shock mode, sustained ventricular fibrillation was induced. This was quickly detected by the device, which charged and delivered a 28-joule biphasic countershock at an impedance of 900 ohms, successfully converting the rhythm to sinus. After waiting 10 minutes, sustained ventricular fibrillation was again induced. At this time, a 29-joule biphasic countershock was successful in converting the rhythm to sinus, at an impedance of 898 ohms. At this time, implant criteria was completed with defibrillation thresholds of less than or equal to 35 joules.

The wound was closed using 2-0 Vicryl in interrupted sutures for the facial layer, 2-0 Vicryl in a running by-layer suture for the subcutaneous layer, and Indermil for the skin layer.

The patient tolerated the procedure well without apparent complications and was transferred to Recovery in stable condition. A chest x-ray was ordered and is pending at the time of this dictation.

CONCLUSION: Successful implantation of transvenous dual chamber defibrillator, with defibrillator thresholds of less than or equal to 35 joules.

Proofreading & Editing Exercise

COMPLEX PERCUTANEOUS INTERVENTION ON PERIPHERAL VASCULATURE

PERIPHERAL INTERVENTION PROCEDURE

PROCEDURE:
1. Antegrade right popliteal artery FoxHollow arthrectomy and angiogram.
2. Antegrade right anterior tibial artery proximal and distal segment rotational arthrectomy with 1.5 and 2.5 mm burs, percutaneous transluminal angioplasty, and angiography.
3. Right proximal dorsalis pedis artery FoxHollow arthrectomy, percutaneous transluminal angioplasty, and angiography.
4. Antegrade left distal posterior tibial artery percutaneous transluminal angioplasty and angiography.

CLINICAL HISTORY:
Patient is a 73-year-old male with a nonhealing foot ulcer.

TECHNIQUE:
Consent was obtained after explaining the risks, benefits, and alternatives, risks involving renal failure, retroperitoneal hemorrhage, bleeding, stroke, distal embolization, and imponderables. With a single stick, access was gained into the right common femoral artery by antegrade technique. We crossed the subtotally occluded anterior tibial artery via a stiff glide wire, which we exchanged over a Quick-Cross catheter to a PT Graphix wire. This was exchanged over a Transit catheter to a RotaWire floppy guide. Nitroglycerin 200 mcg was given to defuse spasm. Angiomax was administered. This was followed by rotational arthrectomy of the anterior tibial artery with a 1.5 mm bur. Multiple cuts were made in the proximal, mid, and distal segments. This resulted in a reduction of stenosis to about 70%. This was followed by rotational arthrectomy with a 2.0 mm bur in the proximal, mid, and distal segments. This was followed by angiogram which revealed slow reflow-no reflow phenomenon. At this time, we administered papaverine 60 mg intraarterially, and gave 200 mcg of nitroglycerin intraarterially. There was slow flow detected. ReoPro intraarterial was administered as well, and a drip started.

At this time, we redirected the wire into the posterior tibial artery. FoxHollow arthrectomy of the popliteal artery was performed. Multiple cuts were made with a large amount of plaque removed. Stenosis was reduced from 70% to less than 20%, with no evidence of any dissection or embolization.

This was followed by PTA of the distal posterior tibial artery with a 2 x 30 mm Maverick balloon. Three inflations were made for 60 and 90 seconds each. Stenosis was reduced from 99% to less than 20%. There was flow seen into the plantar arch; however, there was diffuse, severe disease which was left untouched.

(continued)

At this time, the wire was again redirected into the dorsalis pedis artery. Rotational arthrectomy was performed. This was followed by PTA with a 2.5 x 30 mm Maverick balloon to 6 atmospheres for 90 seconds. Stenosis was reduced to less than 20%. There was no evidence of any dissection or embolization.

NOTE:
This was an extremely complicated, long, drawn-out procedure with good results.

IMPRESSION:
1. Successful FoxHollow arthrectomy of the right popliteal artery.
2. Successful rotational arthrectomy and percutaneous transluminal angioplasty of the ATA.
3. Successful rotational arthrectomy and percutaneous transluminal angioplasty of the proximal dorsalis pedis artery.
4. Successful percutaneous transluminal angioplasty of the left posterior tibial artery distal segment.

PLAN:
At this point, patient has much better flow in his foot, with his wound having its best chance for healing. If this does not heal, we may not have any more interventional options left.

Proofreading & Editing Exercise

CORRECTIVE SURGERY FOR COMPLEX CONGENITAL HEART DEFECTS (PEDIATRIC)

OPERATIVE REPORT

PREOPERATIVE DIAGNOSIS: D-transposition of the great arteries with large perimembranous ventricular septal defect and intramural right coronary artery, status post balloon atrial septostomy.

POSTOPERATIVE DIAGNOSIS: D-transposition of the great arteries with large perimembranous ventricular septal defect and intramural right coronary artery, status post balloon atrial septostomy.

OPERATION: Arterial switch procedure; ventricular septal defect closure using pericardial patch; atrial septal defect closure using pericardial patch; patent ductus arteriosus ligation and division.

SURGEON: XXXX

ASSISTANT: XXXX

ANESTHESIA: General.

INDICATIONS: This 5-day-old, 2200-gm boy was followed in fetal life with transposition of the great vessels and a ventricular septal defect. The baby was born at 37 weeks and was mildly cyanotic. Echocardiography revealed the above diagnosis. There was a large perimembranous ventricular septal defect. There was a right anterior aorta from which two coronary ostia could be seen. The right coronary, however, appeared to empty fairly high in the root, indicating an intramural course. The left gave rise to the circumflex in the anterior facing sinus. Balloon atrial septostomy was performed to stabilize the baby. The baby was then brought to the operating room a few days later for the following procedure.

PROCEDURE: Following induction of amnesia, the baby was sterilely prepped and draped and given IV antibiotics. A midline chest incision was made and carried down through the sternum, and a retractor placed. The thymus gland was incised. The pericardium was cleaned off and a generous patch excised and tanned in glutaraldehyde. Remaining pericardium was opened. The innominate vein was mobilized. Then, the great vessels, including the main pulmonary artery and both branches, were mobilized. The ductus arteriosus was exposed. A pantaloon patch of pulmonary homograft was sawed then trimmed appropriately. Marking sutures of 7-0 Prolene were placed on the matching sinuses for the proposed site of coronary artery transfer. The right coronary artery lacked an ostial bulge, but its intramural course was partially visible as a prominence that went 4 to 5 mm distal and posterior on the anterior root. Heparin, 300 units/kg, was given, then a straight venous cannula was placed in the atrium and angled in the inferior vena cava. An 8-French

(continued)

arterial cannula was placed. Cardiopulmonary bypass was begun with cooling to 18 degrees over 25 minutes. The ductus arteriosus was further dissected out, then ligated on the aortic side with a 2-0 Tevdek tie. A vent was placed through the right pulmonary vein into the left ventricle, tourniquets placed around the cavae; a point of proposed division of the anterior great artery was chosen, and a cardioplegic catheter was placed there. The aorta was occluded with a clamp, and 25 mL/kg of crystalloid cardioplegia was given, with subsequent doses of 10 mL/kg given every 20 to 30 minutes, using an olive-tipped catheter. The right atrial cannula was now advanced into the superior vena cava and secured with a tourniquet, and the inferior caval tourniquet was tightened. An oblique right atriotomy incision was made and traction sutures placed. Through the tricuspid valve, a large perimembranous defect could easily be seen. Traction sutures were placed on the septal leaf, on the anterior leaflet, and then a Tevdek tie placed around some prominent chords of the septal leaflet. With this exposure, the ventricular septal defect was now closed with a pericardial patch and running 7-0 Prolene suture. The tricuspid valve was tested and was competent. The atrial septal defect was large and there was foraminal tissue loss. Therefore, this was closed with a second pericardial patch and running 7-0 Prolene suture. The right atriotomy was then partially closed with running, doubly run 6-0 Prolene suture. A maintenance dose of cardioplegia was given, and the cardioplegic catheter was removed; the aorta was divided at that location. The route was inspected, and the entry point of the right coronary artery could be seen just above the posterior commissure and directly next to it. The left coronary ostium was separate in the anterior sinus, as expected. The ductus arteriosus was now doubly ligated with a 6-0 Prolene pursestring suture, then divided. Then, the main pulmonary artery was divided distal to the marking sutures, near its bifurcation. The branch pulmonary arteries were then completely mobilized with cautery and a LeCompte maneuver performed. A traction suture was placed on the anterior root to bring both roots anteriorly. The coronary ostia were again inspected, then generous buttons cut out, using tenotomy scissors. The right coronary artery required takedown of the posterior commissure of the anterior valve in order to achieve an adequate-size button. Both buttons were then mobilized with low-power cautery and care was taken to preserve all coronary artery branches possible. A U-shaped incision was then made in the matching sinuses, and root tissue was removed to achieve a better circumferential match with the aortic arch. Each coronary was then implanted into its matching location on the posterior root using running 7-0 Maxon suture. Each suture arm was tied to a separately placed 7-0 Maxon stitch. Aorta was then anastomosed to the posterior root using a running 7-0 Maxon suture. At near-completion, the olive-tipped catheter was placed in the aortic root and a dose of cardioplegia given in order to observe coronary filling and general anatomy. The coronaries filled nicely and the anatomy appeared appropriate. Now, the pantaloon pulmonary homograft patch was used to reconstruct the anterior root, resuspending the commissure to the homograft patch. The patch was then trimmed. The patient was placed in partial Trendelenburg and the heart allowed to fill some while de-airing through suture lines. The aortic clamp was then removed. Both coronary systems filled well and the heart began beating in spontaneous sinus rhythm. The pulmonary bifurcation was then anastomosed to the anterior root using a running 7-0 Prolene

(continued)

suture. The ductal tissue on the bifurcation area was extremely friable and de-hissed during placement of the bifurcation sutures. Therefore, in place of all ductal tissue, we replaced the superior portion of the bifurcation area with a separate patch of pulmonary homograft. This assured that both left and right pulmonary branches were wide open and under no tension. Rewarming was started. Suture lines were inspected for hemostasis. A single right atrial catheter was placed and secured to the skin. The pleural cavities were opened and drained of fluid. The caval tourniquets were removed. Milrinone, dopamine and epinephrine were started. The lungs were ventilated. There was good cardiac activity at 36 degrees core temperature and no evidence of coronary ischemia. There were no regional wall motion abnormalities as viewed directly. Cardiopulmonary bypass was then discontinued. The venous cannulas were removed. The hemodynamics were observed, and the right atrial pressure was 8 mmHg with a blood pressure of 65/30, a heart rate of 140 in sinus rhythm, with a narrow QRS complex. The QRS did seem to vary intermittently and suddenly, but with no hemodynamic compromise. There were no arrhythmias. The arterial cannula was therefore removed and protamine sulfate given. All suture lines were packed with thrombin-Gelfoam and Surgicel. Ultimately, good hemostasis was achieved. Surgical glue was then applied to the suture lines. The mediastinum was thoroughly irrigated with antibiotic saline solution. A 16-French drain tube was placed, secured to the skin, and set to feeding tube suction. After a final inspection and confirmation of counts, the chest was closed in layers with interrupted stainless steel wires and layers of running absorbable suture. A dry dressing was placed. The baby tolerated the procedure apparently well, and care was continued in the cardiac intensive care unit.

Proofreading & Editing Exercise

Report #31

TWO-DIMENSIONAL STUDY

CARDIAC NONINVASIVE STUDY

PROCEDURE: Two-dimensional limited study.

INDICATION: This is a 64-year-old with a history of congestive heart failure. This test is being done to evaluate for interventricular dyssynchrony.

TECHNIQUE: This is a 2-D limited study. Ejection fraction appears to be 35%. In evaluating for intraventricular dyssynchrony, the septal to the posterior wall level of the papilla muscle is 120 msec, which is not significant. Tissue Doppler was done of the basil septal wall, basil inferior wall, basil anterior wall, basilar lateral wall. The QRS to the peak systolic velocity of the septal wall is 185 msec; the QRS to the peak systolic velocity of the inferior wall is 190 msec; the QRS to the peak systolic velocity of the anterior wall is 220 msec; the QRS to the peak systolic velocity of the lateral wall is 205 msec. This is not consistent with any significant of intraventricular dyssynchrony.

In evaluating for interventricular dyssynchrony, the aortic ejection delay is 75 msec, the pulmonic ejection delay is 120 msec. This is consistent with some degree of interventricular dyssynchrony.

CONCLUSION:
1. Moderate left ventricular dysfunction, estimated ejection fraction is 35%.
2. No evidence of interventricular dyssynchrony.
3. Evidence of some degree of intraventricular dyssynchrony.

Proofreading & Editing Exercise

PERCUTANEOUS CORONARY INTERVENTION

OPERATIVE REPORT

PROCEDURE:
1. Placement of a guiding catheter in the right coronary artery.
2. Intravascular ultrasound of the right coronary artery.
3. Drug-eluting stent to the right coronary artery.

BRIEF HISTORY: A 71-year-old female with classic anginal symptoms, who underwent diagnostic catheterization preceding this intervention. There was a lesion of uncertain significance on a bend in the proximal right coronary artery, and we are asked to perform intervascular ultrasound and intervention, if needed.

PROCEDURE SUMMARY: A 5-French sheath was exchanged for a 6-French sheath in the right femoral artery. Because of a history of a thrombocytopenia, a bolus of Angiomax was given. A 6-French JR4 guiding catheter with side holes was used to correlate the right coronary artery. Initial angiograms revealed a questionable 60% to 70% lesion on a bend after a conus branch, prior to the right ventricular branch. There was a second bend noted in this artery, felt to be less significant, after the right ventricular branch. A 0.014 Stabilizer wire was advanced distally, and spasm of the artery was noted with wire placement.

Subsequently, intravascular ultrasound was performed with several runs. There appeared to be a 70% to 80% inferior eccentric plaque noted at the area in question, in a very short discreet segment. Decision was then made to proceed with stenting.

A 3 x 13-mm Cypher stent was then deployed at 14 atmospheres. This straightened out the bend and reduced the stenosis to 0%. There was some kinking noted at the end of the stent, at the site of the previously-described lesion, which improved with administration of intracoronary nitroglycerin.

The patient had no chest pain or EKG changes with deployment of the stent. She was started on Plavix at the end of the procedure and transferred to the recovery area.

SUMMARY: Intravascular ultrasound of the right coronary artery revealed a 70% eccentric short lesion, successfully stented with a 3 x 13 Cypher stent.

Proofreading & Editing Exercise

Report #33

INTRACARDIAC ELECTROPHYSIOLOGIC STUDY AND RADIOFREQUENCY CATHETER ABLATION (PEDIATRIC)

ELECTROPHYSIOLOGY REPORT

PROCEDURE: Intracardiac electrophysiologic study and radiofrequency catheter ablation.

INDICATIONS: The patient is a 14-year-old with a history of recurrent SVT. She was referred for electrophysiologic study with the plan for catheter ablation.

PROCEDURE/TECHNIQUE: The patient was brought to the catheterization laboratory and prepped and draped in the usual sterile fashion. She was sedated and intubated by Cardiac Anesthesia. Access was obtained with 5-French and 8-French sheaths in the right femoral vein, two 5-French sheaths in the left femoral vein, and a 6-French sheath in the right internal jugular vein. A 5000-unit bolus of heparin was administered. ACT was monitored on an hourly basis. A 5-French quadripolar catheter was placed in the high right atrial appendage, a 5-French quadripolar catheter was placed in the right ventricular apex, and a 5-French Hisser catheter was placed in the anterior tricuspid groove to record a His bundle electrogram. A 5-French decapolar CS catheter was placed in the coronary sinus to record left-sided electrograms. Mapping and ablation were performed using a Bard D-curved ablation catheter. Baseline measurements were obtained. Atrial and ventricular stimulations were performed. A slow pathway ablation was performed. Repeat atrial and ventricular stimulations were performed. All catheters and sheaths were removed and hemostasis was obtained with Safeguard occlusion device. The patient was transported to the pediatric intensive care unit.

ELECTROPHYSIOLOGIC FINDINGS:

BASELINE MEASUREMENTS: Baseline recording demonstrated sinus rhythm at a cycle length of 629 msec. The A-H interval was 52, with an H-V interval of 42.

ATRIAL PACING: Atrial extrastimuli was placed in a drive train of 500 msec. There was evidence for dual AV node physiology with an A-H jump at 280 msec. Atrial ERP was 500/200. AV node ERP was not encountered. There were no AV node echo beats in the baseline state. Rapid atrial pacing demonstrated AV Wenckebach at 340 msec. Once again, there were no AV node echo beats or inducible SVT in the baseline state. Later in the case, following ventricular pacing, repeat atrial extrastimulus pacing and rapid atrial pacing were performed during Isuprel infusion and Isuprel elimination. During Isuprel elimination, the patient had reproducibly inducible SVT. The SVT had a cycle length of 289 msec with concentric activation in a VA of 18 msec, consistent with AV node reentry tachycardia. This was terminated with burst atrial pacing and, once again, reproducible.

(continued)

VENTRICULAR PACING: Ventricular extrastimuli were placed in a drive train of 500 msec. There was concentric, decremental VA conduction. V ERP was 500/220. VA ERP was not encountered. Rapid ventricular pacing demonstrated VA block at 300 msec. There was no inducible SVT with ventricular pacing protocol. This protocol was repeated during an Isuprel infusion. Once again, there was no inducible SVT.

MAPPING AND ABLATION: Based on electrophysiologic findings, the patient was noted to have SVT due to AV node reentry tachycardia. Therefore, a slow pathway ablation was performed. The ablation catheter was positioned in the posteroseptal space, superior to the os of the coronary sinus. Of note, the coronary sinus so was quite dilated and the positioning was almost toward the mid-septal region. Application of radiofrequency energy was administered while there was a small atrial electrogram and a large ventricular electrogram. Initially, there was junctional acceleration where the atrial signals preceded the ventricular signals. The peak temperature during this lesion was approximately 54 degrees. The catheter was repositioned somewhat more superiorly. Repeat radiofrequency energy was administered for a total of 40 seconds, with a peak temperature of 56 degrees. During this time, there was junctional acceleration with 1:1 VA conduction.

POSTABLATION TESTING: Following slow pathway ablation, the patient was in sinus rhythm with normal AV conduction. Atrial extrastimulus pacing and rapid atrial pacing were performed in the baseline state, during Isuprel infusion, and during Isuprel elimination. This was repeated with two cycles of Isuprel infusion and Isuprel elimination, with repeat testing. The maximum response with very rapid atrial pacing was a single echo beat, with no inducible SVT.

IMPRESSION: Supraventricular tachycardia due to atrioventricular node reentry tachycardia. Acutely successful slow pathway ablation.

PLAN: The patient will be monitored in the pediatric intensive care unit. She will undergo an ECG and echocardiogram. Followup will be with her routine cardiologist in approximately 2 weeks.

Proofreading & Editing Exercise   Report #34

TRANSESOPHAGEAL ECHOCARDIOGRAM

CARDIOLOGY PROCEDURE REPORT

PROCEDURE: Transesophageal electrocardiogram.

INDICATIONS: An 81-year-old with weakness of the legs; study is ordered to evaluate for source of embolus.

TECHNIQUE: The transesophageal echocardiogram was performed without difficulty. Sedation was given in the form of 1 mg of Versed and 12.5 mg Demerol; the patient was adequately sedated with these dosages. Following probe placement, the overall LV function was evaluated and was 65%. There was evidence of a trace effusion noted. The aortic valve appeared to be trileaflet and slightly sclerotic, with Lamb excrescences seen, with trace aortic regurgitation noted. The mitral valve appeared to be apparently normal, with no mitral regurgitation. Trace tricuspid insufficiency was noted, with normal tricuspid valve. The pulmonary valve was well visualized and appeared to have mild pulmonic insufficiency. There was mild plaque seen of the aortic root. There was no evidence of ASD or VSD. The atrial appendage was well visualized and had no apparent clot.

CONCLUSION: Preserved left ventricular function. Slight sclerosis of the aortic valve, with trace aortic insufficiency seen. There appears to be trace pericardial effusion. Mild pulmonic insufficiency is seen. Aortic valve has Lamb excrescences. In the ascending portion, there was some mild plaque seen in the aortic root, but there did not appear to be any thrombogenic material that would suggest a source of embolus. Overall ejection fraction was 60%.

Proofreading & Editing Exercise

Report #35

LOWER EXTREMITY GRAFT IMAGING STUDY

VASCULAR IMAGING STUDY

TEST PERFORMED:
Lower extremity graft imaging study.

INDICATIONS:
The patient is a 61-year-old man with a right-to-left femorofemoral crossover graft and a left femoral-posterior tibial bypass graft, using composite arm veins. This is a surveying study.

Imaging of the left leg shows a widely patent graft down to just above the distal anastomosis where there is a velocity acceleration of 590 cm/second.

IMPRESSION:
Widely patient left femoral-posterior tibial bypass except for a high-grade stenosis of the graft just above the distal anastomosis.

Proofreading & Editing Exercise

RIGHT GROIN IMAGING STUDY

VASCULAR IMAGING STUDY

STUDY TITLE
Right groin imaging study.

INDICATIONS
The patient is a 22-year-old man status post shotgun wound to the lateral aspect of the right thigh. This is a follow-up study of the right common femoral artery and vein.

STUDY
Imaging of the right medial thigh shows no evidence of an arterial or venous false aneurysm or fistula. There is no evidence of a deep venous thrombosis in the veins. Multiple shotgun pellets are seen.

IMPRESSION
There does not appear to be any injury to the arteries or veins in this area, nor any evidence of a venous thrombosis.

Proofreading & Editing Exercise

Report #37

PACEMAKER GENERATOR REPLACEMENT

PACEMAKER REPORT

PROCEDURE IN DETAIL: The patient was prepped in the usual sterile fashion. The right previous pacer site was in the right subclavian area. An incision was made. The pulse generator was removed. The ventricular lead was checked. Sensitivity was 5.8 mV, voltage 1.3 V, 2.4 mA, resistance 450 ohms. The same pacemaker pocket was used. A pulse generator (Affinity SR, serial number XXXXXX) was placed. The patient was sutured in the usual sterile fashion. The patient tolerated the procedure well.

Proofreading & Editing Exercise

ELECTRICAL CARDIOVERSION

CARDIOLOGY PROCEDURE REPORT

PROCEDURE: Electrical cardioversion.

INDICATIONS: A 70-year-old, status post aortic valve replacement, thoracic aortic aneurysm repair with aortic valve conduct, and reimplantation of the coronary arteries, postoperatively has developed episodes of atrial fibrillation, atrial flutter, and atrial tachycardia.

On preconversion electrocardiogram, the patient's rhythm showed what may be in ectopic atrial tachycardia with a ventricular rate of 100 beats per minute, with a right bundle branch block pattern. We proceeded to perform synchronized electrical cardioversion.

SEDATION: Versed 2 mg and 30 mg of Diprivan.

TECHNIQUE: Once adequate sedation was obtained, synchronized electrical cardioversion was performed with 20 jewels.

Postconversion electrocardiogram shows well-defined atrial wave which is probably a sinus wave, with marked first-degree AV block. The other possibility is that this is a low atrial rhythm, end-conducted with first degree AV block. Flutter P waves are not identified.

The patient tolerated the procedure well.

Proofreading & Editing Exercise

Report #39

M-MODE, TWO-DIMENSIONAL ECHOCARDIOGRAM WITH COLOR FLOW DOPPLER

ECHOCARDIOGRAM

PROCEDURE: M-mode, two dimensional echocardiogram with color flow Doppler.

INDICATION: Cardiac mass.

Left atrial cavity is mildly dilated, measuring approximately 4.2 cm. Mitral annular valve is mildly calcified. The aortic root is normal. The aortic valve leaflets are normal with normal leaflet extrusion. Ventricular cavity is mildly dilated, with global hypokinesia, and overall ejection fraction measuring 25%. There is a mobile mass present at the apex of the heart which appears to be a thrombus. This mass measures approximately 7 mm. The right atrium and right ventricular cavity are mildly dilated. No pericardial effusion is present. Doppler shows the presence of mild mitral and tricuspid regurgitation.

CONCLUSION:
1. Cardiomyopathy with reduced ejection fraction of 25%.
2. Apical thrombus measuring 7 mm.
3. Mild mitral regurgitation.
4. Mild tricuspid regurgitation.
5. No pericardial effusion.

Proofreading & Editing Exercise

Report #40

ECHOCARDIOGRAM

ECHOCARDIOGRAM STUDY

FINDINGS:

1. Technically adequate study. Rhythm is irregular.

2. The echocardiographic appearance of the aortic valve is a normal-appearing semilunar valve with adequate excursion. There is mild aortic root sclerosis. The aortic root is of normal dimension. Mitral valve is mildly thickened with mildly decreased opening felt secondary to low cardiac output. Tricuspid and pulmonic valves was suboptimally imaged but appeared grossly normal.

3. Left atrium is moderately enlarged. Left ventricle is moderately dilated as well. Right atrium and right ventricle appear to be at upper limits of normal in dimensions.

4. The left ventricular wall thickness appears to be at upper limits of normal. The basal inferior segment is akinetic. Overall left ventricular contractility is moderately to severely impaired, with the ejection fraction estimated at 20% to 25%. Right ventricular contractility is moderately impaired.

5. No intracavitary mass, thrombus or valvular vegetations are identified.

6. No pericardial effusion is present.

7. Doppler reveals mild mitral regurgitation. There is increased E:A ratio, consistent with a restricted pattern of diastolic dysfunction. There is mild tricuspid regurgitation also present.

CONCLUSIONS:

1. Dilated cardiomyopathy with mildly dilated left ventricle and moderately dilated left atrium present. Severe global wall motion abnormalities as described above with severely impaired left ventricular systolic function. Impaired right ventricular function is also seen.

2. Fibrocalsific changes of the aortic and mitral valve without significant valvular disease.

3. Mild mitral and tricuspid regurgitation.

Proofreading & Editing Exercise

ABNORMAL ELECTROPHYSIOLOGIC STUDY

ELECTROPHYSIOLOGIC STUDY

PROCEDURE:

Electrophysiologic study.

CLINICAL HISTORY:

Syncope.

PROCEDURE/TECHNIQUE:

After informed consent was obtained, the patient was brought to the laboratory in a fasting state. He was prepped and draped in the usual sterile fashion with Betadine scrub and pain. Local infiltration with Polocaine 1% was used to achieve anesthesia. Using a #18-gauge needle, access was obtained into the right femoral vein. Over a guide wire, a 6-French sheath was advanced into this vessel. Using identical technique at 2 sites along the course of the right femoral vein, and through these sheaths, three 5-French, 5-mm quadripolar electrode catheters were advanced using fluoroscopic guidance. These 5-French, 5-mm quadripolar electrode catheters were advanced to positions in the high right atrium, right ventricular apex, and to a position across the tricuspid annulus such that a His bundle electrogram could be carefully mapped and recorded. After baseline intervals and pacing thresholds were obtained, RA and RV incremental pacing and programmed stimulation were performed. Sinus node recovery times were performed. Carotid sinus massage was performed. Gentle left-sided carotid sinus massage was associated with a systole of 6.5 seconds, a reproducible finding. At the end of the procedure, all catheters and sheaths were removed. He tolerated the procedure well.

FINDINGS:

1. At baseline, intracardiac intervals are normal with an AH interval of 50 msec and an HV interval of 54 msec.
2. Sinus node function is normal. All sinus node and all corrected sinus node recovery times are within normal limits. The longest corrected sinus node recovery time is normal at 166 msec.
3. AV nodal function is normal with an antegrade Wenckebach cycle length of 380 msec and an AV nodal refractory period of 550/300.
4. No supraventricular arrhythmias were inducible.
5. Ventricular tachycardia is not inducible during this procedure, even with very aggressive pacing protocols. This includes RV incremental pacing and programmed stimulation at 2 sites, with 2 drive cycle lengths and up to 3 extra stimuli.
6. Marked carotid hypersensitivity is noted, with episodes of a systole of 6.5 seconds.

(continued)

CONCLUSION:

This study is remarkable for marked carotid hypersensitivity with episodes of a systole associated with hypotension and a supine blood pressure of 75 mmHg.

RECOMMENDATIONS:

Given these findings, will recommend permanent pacemaker implantation.

Proofreading & Editing Exercise   Report #42

TRANSLUMINAL ANGIOPLASTY AND ANGIOGRAPHY

VASCULAR INTERVENTIONAL PROCEDURE

PROCEDURE:

1. Right axillary artery percutaneous transluminal angioplasty and angiogram.
2. Right common iliac artery percutaneous transluminal angioplasty and angiogram.
3. Unsuccessful right common femoral artery percutaneous transluminal angioplasty and angiogram.

CLINICAL HISTORY:

Patient is a 77-year-old female with bilateral leg claudication, right worse than the left.

TECHNIQUE:

Consent was obtained after explaining the risks, benefits, and alternatives, risks involving renal failure, retroperitoneal hemorrhage, bleeding, stroke, and imponderables. Single-stick access was gained in the right brachial artery. A 5-French sheath was placed. At this time, we tried to pass a wire into the subclavian artery, however, we could not make it pass into the artery at this time. Angiogram revealed a 70% focal short stenosis of the axillary artery. At this time, we placed a glide wire across the stenosis in the right axillary artery. This was followed by PTA with a 5 x 40 OPTA PRO balloon. It was inflated to 10 atmospheres for 90 seconds; stenosis was reduced from 70% to 20% with no evidence of dissection or embolization. Prior to this, Angiomax had been administered.

At this time, with the help of a LIMA catheter and a glide wire, we gained access into the distal abdominal aorta. We switched to a 0.035 non-glide J wire and placed a 90-mm Brite Tip sheath from the right side to the left distal abdominal aorta. With the help of a 5-French angled glide catheter and straight glide wire, and with great difficulty due to extreme tortuosity, we were able to gain access into the common femoral artery. Over a Quick Cross catheter, we placed a straight wire into the superficial femoral artery; however, at this time the Quick Cross catheter got stuck in the struts which were in the right femoral artery from before, which had a residual 40% to 50% stenosis. We had no luck in retrieving the catheter after multiple attempts.

Following that, we gained access into the right common iliac artery after dilating with a 5-French dilator. We were able to place a 7-French, 35-mm Brite Tip sheath into the common iliac artery. We placed a J wire into the distal abdominal aorta. This was followed by PTA of the common iliac artery with a 7 x 40 OPTA PRO balloon to 10 atmospheres for 60 seconds. The balloon was withdrawn. Angiogram revealed

(continued)

persistent 30% residual stenosis. At this time, we were able to successfully retrieve that Quick Cross catheter intact, with nothing embolized distally.

We decided to stop and recommend surgery for her right common femoral artery stenosis.

IMPRESSION:

1. Successful percutaneous transluminal angioplasty of the right axillary artery and right common femoral artery.
2. Unsuccessful percutaneous transluminal angioplasty of the right common femoral artery.

PLAN:

At this point, I would recommend patient undergo patch angioplasty of the right common femoral artery with a femorofemoral bypass surgery.

Proofreading & Editing Exercise

CARDIAC CATHETERIZATION WITH VEIN GRAFT AND LEFT INTERNAL MAMMARY GRAFT ANGIOGRAPHY

OPERATIVE REPORT

TITLE OF PROCEDURE:
1. Left heart catheterization.
2. Coronary angiography.
3. Left ventriculography.
4. Saphenous vein graft angiography.
5. Left internal mammary graft anglography.

PROCEDURE IN DETAIL:
After informed consent was obtained and premedications administered, the area of the right femoral triangle was prepped and draped in the usual sterile fashion. Xylocaine 1% was used for local anesthesia. Modified seldinger technique was used to place a 6-French Hemaquet in the right femoral artery. Using standard Judkins technique with a JL4 and JR4, left followed by right coronary angiography was performed in multiple right anterior oblique and left anterior oblique views. The right coronary catheter was used for angiography of the internal mammary. A multipurpose catheter was used for right coronary artery saphenous vein graft angiography. Finally, a pigtail catheter was used for left ventriculography performed in the 30-degree RAO view. VasoSeal was used for hemostasis. The patient tolerated the procedure well. There were no complications.

The patient remained in a sinus rhythm. Left ventricular end-diastolic pressure was 16. There was no gradient between the left ventricle and aorta on pullback. Left ventriculography revealed mild global hypokinesis but low normal left ventricular systolic function.

CORONARY ANGIOGRAPHY:
Injection of the left coronary system demonstrates a left main which trifurcates into an LAD, ramus and circumflex. Left main has a concentric 60% to 70% distal narrowing involving the trifurcation of the LAD, ramus and circumflex. There is no damping or ventricularization with catheter engagement.

The LAD is a fair-caliber vessel which gives rise to a moderate-size proximal diagonal and multiple septal perforating branches, and the LAD terminates just at the inferior aspect of the left ventricular apex. There is competitive spilling from the mid to distal LAD via the internal mammary bypass. The mid to distal LAD is widely patent and of fair-caliber. There is luminal irregularity in the proximal LAD with no obstructive lesions. Likewise, the first diagonal has diffuse irregularity but no obstructive disease.

The ramus is of smaller caliber and free of obstructive disease.

The right coronary artery is dominant and completely occluded near its origin.

(continued)

SAPHENOUS VEIN GRAFT TO THE POSTERIOR DESCENDING ARTERY:
This graft is widely patent, briskly filling a fair-caliber PDA and a larger posterolateral system. There is some mild luminal irregularity but no obstructive disease in this system.

Proofreading & Editing Exercise

CORONARY ARTERY BYPASS GRAFT

OPERATIVE REPORT

TITLE OF PROCEDURE: Coronary artery bypass graft (CABG).

PROCEDURE IN DETAIL: The patient was brought to the operating room and given general endotracheal anesthesia. The pulmonary artery catheter was inserted by Anesthesia under sterile technique in the right internal jugular vein. The distal right saphenous vein was harvested from the medial malleolus to just above the knee using multiple small serial incisions with skin bridges. It was a good-quality vein. The leg was closed in layers with 2-0 and 3-0 Vicryl, with 3-0 Vicryl subcuticular suture in the skin.

A midline sternotomy was performed. The patient was heparinized. The ascending aorta was found to be extremely calcified after opening the pericardium. There was diffuse atherosclerosis with visible plaque emanating from the ascending aorta. The aortic arch was cannulated beyond the ascending aorta. The atrium was cannulated, and the patient was placed on bypass. A vent was inserted into the left ventricle via the right superior pulmonary vein. Coronaries were marked for bypass, including a very large posterior descending artery and a good-sized posterolateral branch just prior to its bifurcation with two smaller branches. A single-clamp technique was utilized. The aorta was crossclamped in the least calcified place. One liter of cardioplegia was given antegrade to arrest the heart. It was packed with ice and then flushed posteriorly.

Bypasses were accomplished, first using the reverse saphenous vein in an end-to-side fashion to the PDA, which was a good-quality 2.5 to 3-mm vessel. This was done with a reverse vein and running 7-0 Prolene suture. The second bypass was to the posterolateral branch, which was smaller but easily took a 1.5-mm probe. This was done with a separate piece of vein and a running 7-0 Prolene suture. A bolus of cold cardioplegia was given, and the patient was rewarmed. With the crossclamp still in place, a single aortotomy was made in the ascending aorta. The area was thickened and calcified but had a decent lumen to allow suture of the proximal end of the PDA up to the ascending aorta with running 5-0 Prolene suture in an end-to-side fashion. After concluding this anastomosis, hot cardioplegia was given into the aortic root. The crossclamp was removed after a total of 30 minutes crossclamp time. The remaining proximal anastomosis of the posterolateral branch was brought onto the hood of the PDA graft. The PDA was isolated with bulldog clamps. Venotomy was made, and the end-to-side anastomosis of the posterior left ventricle to the PDA was accomplished using running 6-0 Prolene suture in an end-to-side fashion. The system was back bled and de-aired, and the bulldog clamps were removed. Vessels were inspected, and they were both hemostatic.

(continued)

2 atrial and 2 ventricular pacing wires were placed and brought out through the skin. One single chest tube was placed into the mediastinum. Neither pleura was opened. The left ventricular vent was clamped and removed, and the pursestring was ligated. The lungs were inflated. The patient was ventilated and weaned off bypass successfully without the aid of inotropic support. Protamine was started and the atrial cannula was removed. Volume status was normalized and the heparin fully reversed with protamine. The aortic cannula was removed and the site ligated and reinforced with pledgeted 4-0 Prolene stitch. The chest tube was positioned. The wound was closed using figure-of-eight 0 Ethibond to reapproximate fascia, 7 sternal wires, and 2 layers of running 2-0 Vicryl and a running 3-0 Vicryl in the skin. The patient tolerated the procedure and was transferred to the intensive care unit in stable condition.

Proofreading & Editing Exercise

DISCHARGE SUMMARY FOR ISCHEMIC CARDIOMYOPATHY

DISCHARGE SUMMARY

FINAL DIAGNOSES:
1. Ischemic cardiomyopathy
2. Status post defibrillator implantation
3. Ventricular tachycardia in 2004
4. History of amiodarone intolerance
5. Multiple defibrillator shocks
6. Hypertension
7. Hyperlipidemia
8. Status post initiation of mexiletine therapy for suppression of recurrent ventricular tachycardia that had resulted in shocks

HOSPITAL COURSE: The patient was transferred from an outlying hospital due to multiple defibrillator shocks. He underwent loading on mexiletine after initially being placed on amiodarone. Amiodarone was discontinued due to a history of previous intolerance, including symptoms that were thought to be compatible with neuropathy. He tolerated loading with mexiletine well and was tested today, with excellent defibrillation thresholds.

DISCHARGE INSTRUCTIONS: He will be discharged and will followed up with us in approximately 3 months.

DISCHARGE MEDICATIONS: Mexiletine 150 mg p.o. b.i.d. with meals, Plavix 75 mg p.o. q.d., aspirin 325 mg q.d., Vasotec 5 mg b.i.d., Toprol-XL 50 mg b.i.d., Lanoxin 0.25 mg q.d., and folic acid 1 mg q.d.

Proofreading & Editing Exercise

Report #46

AORTIC ARCH ANGIOGRAPHY

VASCULAR IMAGING STUDY

PROCEDURE: Aortic arch angiography, selective bilateral carotid angiography with cerebral angiography. Selective bilateral vertebral angiography with cerebral angiography. Angio-Seal deployment.

IDENTIFYING DATA: Patient is a 65-year-old Hispanic female with noninvasive evidence of high-grade stenosis at the origin of the right internal carotid artery.

DESCRIPTION: After informed consent was obtained, the patient was brought to the catheterization laboratory where the right groin was sterilely prepped and draped, and then anesthetized with Xylocaine. A 5-French sheath was placed in the RFA. An aortic arch angiogram was performed using a 5-French pigtail catheter. A 5-French angled glide catheter was then advanced to the right common carotid artery using an angled 0.035 glide wire. Selective carotid angiography was performed. Straight-lateral and AP-cranial cerebral angiograms were obtained during right carotid injection. The catheter was then redirected into the origin of the right vertebral artery, and right vertebral angiography was obtained. A posterior cerebral angiogram was obtained during right vertebral injection. Catheter was redirected into the left common carotid artery, and left carotid angiography was performed in multiple views. Straight-lateral and AP-cranial cerebral angiograms were obtained during left carotid injection. The catheter was then manipulated into the origin of the left vertebral artery. Left vertebral angiography was obtained. Posterior circulation cerebral angiography was obtained in the AP-cranial view. The catheter was removed. A 6-French Angio-Seal device was deployed, with satisfactory hemostasis.

COMPLICATIONS: None.

FLUOROSCOPY TIME: 5.3 minutes.

CONTRAST: 115 mL.

RESULTS:
1. Aortic arch angiography: The aortic arch is unremarkable. The common carotid arteries appear normal. The right innominate artery, right subclavian artery, as well as left subclavian artery, all appear normal. Vertebral arteries are patent bilaterally with the left vertebral artery appearing larger than the right.
2. Carotid angiography: The right internal carotid artery has a 95% osteal stenosis. The external carotid is normal. The left internal carotid artery has 40% to 50% osteal stenosis. There is 90% osteal stenosis of the left external carotid artery.
3. Vertebral angiography: The vertebral arteries are normal bilaterally.
4. Cerebral angiography: The anterior, middle, and posterior cerebral arteries all appear normal bilaterally. Posterior circulation is intact, with filling more from the

(continued)

left vertebral then from the right vertebral. No occlusive disease or aneurysm was identified.

FINAL IMPRESSION: Critical 95% stenosis at the origin of the right internal carotid artery. There is moderate 50% stenosis at the origin of the left internal carotid artery. Incidental note is made of left external carotid artery stenosis. Cerebral angiogram is unremarkable.

PLAN: Vascular surgical consultation, to access for revascularization.

Proofreading & Editing Exercise

Report #47

RADIOFREQUENCY ABLATION

ELECTROPHYSIOLOGY INTERVENTION STUDY

PROCEDURE: Radiofrequency ablation.

CLINICAL HISTORY: A very pleasant 74-year-old woman with very rapid response to atrial fibrillation that has been refractory to aggressive attempts at antiarrhythmic management including Rythmol, Tambocor, amiodarone. She is aware of the risks, benefits and alternatives to proceeding with radiofrequency ablation and subsequent permanent pacemaker implantation during the electrophysiologic study. She understands and wishes to proceed.

TECHNIQUE: After informed consent was obtained, patient was brought to the electrophysiology laboratory in a fasting state. She was prepped and draped in the usual sterile fashion with multiple layers of Betadine. Lidocaine 1% infiltration was used to achieve local anesthesia in the right inguinal area. Using a #18-gauge needle, access was obtained into the left femoral vein. Over a guide wire, a 6-French sheath was advanced into this vessel. Using identical technique at a separate site along the course of the right femoral vein, a 7-French sheath was advanced. Through these sheaths, a 5-French 5-mm quadripolar electrode catheter was advanced to a position in the right ventricular apex, and a 7-French 2.5-mm Cordis Webster D-curve mapping/ablation catheter was advanced to a position across the tricuspid annulus such that a His bundle electrogram could be carefully mapped and recorded. After baseline intervals and pacing thresholds were obtained, excessive endocardial mapping was performed in the region of the His bundle. Radiofrequency energy was then applied at the site of His bundle activation. This was associated with purposeful induction of iatrogenic complete heart block, with a junctional escape rhythm at 40. The patient was observed for some time and then started on an isoproterenol infusion, after which the above process was repeated. No AV conduction was present. The patient continued to have a junctional escape rhythm at 40. Temporary pacing was accomplished to the right ventricular lead until a permanent pacemaker, which had previously been scheduled, could be implanted. He tolerated the procedure quite well.

CONCLUSION: Successful radiofrequency ablation.

Will proceed with previously scheduled permanent pacemaker.

Proofreading & Editing Exercise

CARDIAC CATHETERIZATION WITH PUMP INSERTION AND PACEMAKER WIRE INSERTION

PACEMAKER REPORT

FINAL DIAGNOSES:
1. severe 3-vessel coronary artery disease
2. acute anterior subendocardial myocardial infarction
3. mild to moderate left ventricular systolic dysfunction

PROCEDURES PERFORMED:
1. cardiac catheterization
2. selective coronary arteriography
3. left ventriculography
4. intraaortic balloon pump insertion
5. temporary transvenous pacemaker wire insertion

INDICATIONS: This patient has acute subendocardial myocardial infarction.

DESCRIPTION OF PROCEDURE: The patient was prepped and draped in the usual sterile fashion. Versed 1 mg IV conscious sedation was given. Local anesthesia was then applied to the right groin. An 8-French sheath was placed in the right femoral artery without difficulty. A 6-French sheath was then placed in the right femoral vein without difficulty. The 6-French JL4 and 6-French JR4 diagnostic catheters were used to perform selective coronary arteriography in various LAO and RAO projections. Left ventriculogram in the RAO projection was then performed by advancing a pigtail catheter into the left ventricle. Continuous pressure monitoring was performed during pullback of this catheter across the aortic valve. Upon identification of the anatomy, an intraaortic balloon pump was inserted, and a temporary transvenous pacemaker wire was inserted.

LEFT MAIN: The left main coronary artery is a large-caliper vessel with minimal irregularities.

LEFT ANTERIOR DESCENDING: The LAD is a large-caliber vessel that gives rise to a moderate-sized first diagonal branch and small second diagonal branch. Following the origin of the first diagonal branch, there is a long 90% to 95% stenosis. There are filling defects within this lesion consistent with thrombus. The remainder of the mid LAD and distal LAD has some mild diffuse disease. The first diagonal branch has a proximal 40% stenosis and mild, diffuse disease. The second diagonal branch is a small vessel with a proximal 70% stenosis.

LEFT CIRCUMFLEX: The left circumflex coronary artery is a large, nondominant vessel. It is ectatic in appearance and gives rise to a moderate-sized first marginal branch and moderate-sized second bifurcating marginal branch. The second marginal branch

(continued)

has a 60% stenosis in both limbs of the bifurcation and mild, diffuse disease. The reminder of the circumflex has mild to moderate diffuse disease.

RIGHT CORONARY ARTERY: The RCA is a large, dominant vessel. It gives rise to a moderate-sized posterolateral branch and a moderate-sized posterior descending branch. In the mid right coronary artery there is a 40% eccentric stenosis. The ostium of the posterior descending artery is then narrowed by approximately 90%. The remainder of the PDA has only minimal irregularities.

LEFT VENTRICULOGRAM: Left ventricular systolic function is mildly to moderately diminished. Estimated ejection fraction is 40%. There is anterolateral severe hypokinesis. There is no mitral regurgitation. There is no gradient across the aortic valve. Left ventricular end-diastolic pressure is 22.

DEVICE INSERTION: Upon identification of the anatomy, the 8-French right femoral arterial sheath was exchanged for an 8-French balloon pump sheath. A 40-mL intraaortic balloon pump was then inserted in the usual fashion. A 5-French pacemaker wire was advanced through the right femoral venous sheath to the right ventricular apex and was tested. Testing of thresholds revealed threshold to be less than 0.5 mA. The pacemaker was then set for a backup rate of 40.

COMMENTS: Based on the patient's anatomy, a decision is made for the patient to undergo surgical revascularization. The cardiothoracic surgeon came to the catheterization laboratory and reviewed the images. He agreed this was a suitable strategy for the patient. Because the patient had received Plavix and Integrilin, it was felt that surgery should be delayed a period of hours to days to reduce bleeding risk. For that reason, an intraaortic balloon pump was inserted. Given what we believe is a new left anterior fascicular block and right bundle branch block, a temporary transvenous pacemaker wire was inserted.

Proofreading & Editing Exercise

Report #49

INSERTION OF TRANSVENOUS TEMPORARY PACEMAKER

PACEMAKER REPORT

TITLE OF PROCEDURE: Insertion of transvenous temporary pacemaker by right internal jugular route.

PROCEDURE IN DETAIL: A right jugular stick following Xylocaine anesthesia was made in the triangle between the medial and lateral heads of the trapezius muscles. The internal jugular vein was cannulated initially with needles, using a guidewire. An Arrow introducer sheath was placed. The transvenous pacemaker selected was 3-French. The introducer sheath required a 5-French catheter to maintain a good seal. Intravenous fluid was infused via the side ports of the catheter following good venous return.

The transvenous balloon-type catheter, a flow-directed catheter but without capability of hemodynamic monitoring, was inserted with balloon up to approximately 45 cm and then manipulated between 52 cm from the introducer up to 32 cm from the introducer with best capture seen at 32 cm. Partial capturing was seen at settings at 0.5 mA to 1 mA with good capture at 2 mA. The rate was set at 60 beats per minute with complete capturing. Steri-Strips were used to wrap around the external portion of the catheter, and the catheter was secured to the introducer site port tubing. X-ray was taken showing the tip of the catheter within the right ventricle in good position.

Proofreading & Editing Exercise

Report #50

IMPLANTATION OF CARDIOVERTER DEFIBRILLATOR

CARDIOLOGY PROCEDURE REPORT

PROCEDURES:
1. Implantation of an implantable cardioverter defibrillator.
2. Defibrillation threshold testing.
3. Final programming of the device.

PREPROCEDURE DIAGNOSIS: Ventricular tachycardia.

POSTPROCEDURE DIAGNOSIS: Ventricular tachycardia.

ANESTHESIA: Diprivan.

COMPLICATIONS: None.

DEFIBRILLATOR GENERATOR: Guidant Ventak Mini IV model #1790, serial #XXXXXX.

DEFIBRILLATOR LEAD: Intermedics model #497-23-70, serial #XXXXX, single-coil defibrillator lead.

BRIEF HISTORY: The patient is a 64-year-old white male who has a history of ischemic cardiomyopathy. he had ventricular tachycardia preoperatively and was found to have triple-vessel coronary disease. He underwent six-vessel bypass surgery and underwent postoperative electrophysiologic study which revealed reliably induced ventricular fibrillation with his developing sustained monomorphic ventricular tachycardia after infusion of intravenous procainamide. Because of this, it was recommended that a defibrillator be placed.

PROCEDURE: After informed consent was signed, the patient was brought to the electrophysiology laboratory, and the left infraclavicular area was prepped and draped in the usual sterile fashion. The area was infused with 1% Xylocaine, and a defibrillator pocket was formed with the incision made parallel from the left clavicle down to the level of the prepectoral fascia. The left subclavian vein was then easily cannulated, and over a guidewire a 10.5-French sheath was passed without difficulty. Through this sheath an Intermedics model #497-23-70 single coil tined defibrillator lead was passed under fluoroscopic guidance to the left ventricular apex.

After adequate endocardial anchoring, threshold testing via the pacing system analyzer ensued: R waves measured 5.6 mV, ventricular capture down to an amplitude of 0.5 V, and a pulse width of 0.5 msec, measuring a current of 1.2 mA. The final volt resistance measured 400 ohms. Since these were felt to be appropriate pacing-sensing thresholds, the lead was anchored using the anchoring sleeve with two 2-0 Ethibond sutures. After this, the lead was attached to a CPI/Guidant Ventak Mini IV, model #1790, serial #XXXXXX, defibrillator. The defibrillator was set to detect ventricular fibrillation for any heart rate exceeding 180 beats per minute.

(continued)

Once attached, R waves measured 6.3 mV, impedance measured 416 ohms, and capture was less than 0.6 V, indicating appropriate connections.

The defibrillator and additional lead were then placed in the free-form pocket, and defibrillation threshold testing ensued:

Test #1: Using shock on T-wave algorithm, ventricular fibrillation was induced, and after 9.3 seconds a 17-joule shock was delivered which converted the arrhythmia to normal sinus rhythm. The shock impedance measured 88 ohms.

Test #2: Using similar simulation, ventricular fibrillation was induced, and after 8.8 seconds another 17-joule shock was delivered which promptly converted ventricular fibrillation to normal sinus rhythm. The shock impedance measured 82 ohms. These were felt to be appropriate responses with adequate impedances.

The defibrillator was left in position. The pocket was closed with two layers of 3-0 Vicryl sutures to the subcutaneous tissues and a single layer of 4-0 Vicryl sutures using a subcuticular stitch. Steri-Strips and a pressure dressing were then applied.

The patient was awaken from anesthesia and tolerated the procedure well. She was transferred to the progressive care unit in stable condition.

CONCLUSIONS:
1. Successful implantation of a CPI Mini IV transvenous defibrillator and Intermedics single-coil ventricular lead.
2. Defibrillation threshold less than or equal to 17 joules.
3. Reliably induced ventricular fibrillation.
4. Final programming as mentioned above with the first shock energy set at 27 joules.

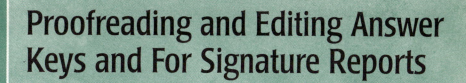

Proofreading and Editing Answer Keys and For Signature Reports

Terminology and Abbreviations Used in the Proofreading and Editing Answer Keys

The terms and abbreviations below are used throughout the Proofreading and Editing Answer Keys to succinctly provide feedback and remediation.

Feedback	Meaning
alt.	acceptable alternative
NOTE	helpful information that does not necessitate a change to the report
s/b	"should be"
spell out	write out the full term instead of using an abbreviation

Sources for Grammar, Style and Usage Rules	Refers To
AAMT Book of Style	The AAMT Book of Style for Medical Transcription, 2nd Edition
ISMP List of Dangerous Abbreviations	The Institute for Safe Medication Practices List of Dangerous Abbreviations
Stedman's Medical Dictionary, 28E	Stedman's Medical Dictionary, 28th Edition

Answer Key

CAROTID DUPLEX SCAN

CAROTID IMAGING

NAME OF TEST: Carotid duplex scan.

INDICATIONS: ~~The patient is a~~ 77 year old man with a known occlusion of the right internal carotid artery and a left carotid artery bypass.

RIGHT CAROTID ARTERY: The internal carotid is occluded. The common and external carotid arteries are widely patent.

LEFT CAROTID ARTERY: The bypass graft from the common to the internal carotid is widely patent. The external carotid appears to be occluded.

VERTEBRAL FLOW: Antegrade on the right and auscultatory ~~on~~ the left.

IMPRESSION:

Occlusion of the right internal carotid artery. Widely patent left carotid bypass. Auscultatory flow in the left vertebral artery is suggestive a left subclavian steel syndrome.

Margin annotations:

insert hyphens to connect an adjectival phrase describing a noun, AAMT Book of Style, ages

move to same line as heading for format continuity

insert *of,* missing word

s/b *oscillatory,* incorrect word, Stedman's Medical Dictionary, 28E

s/b *steal,* incorrect spelling, Stedman's Cardiovascular & Pulmonary Words, 4E

For Signature

CAROTID DUPLEX SCAN

CAROTID IMAGING

NAME OF TEST: Carotid duplex scan.

INDICATIONS: The patient is a 77-year-old man with a known occlusion of the right internal carotid artery and a left carotid artery bypass.

RIGHT CAROTID ARTERY: The internal carotid is occluded. The common and external carotid arteries are widely patent.

LEFT CAROTID ARTERY: The bypass graft from the common to the internal carotid is widely patent. The external carotid appears to be occluded.

VERTEBRAL FLOW: Antegrade on the right and oscillatory on the left.

IMPRESSION: Occlusion of the right internal carotid artery. Widely patent left carotid bypass. Oscillatory flow in the left vertebral artery is suggestive of a left subclavian steal syndrome.

Answer Key

DEATH SUMMARY

CLINICAL RESUME

FINAL DIAGNOSIS:

1. Status post acute anterior wall myocardial infarction with left ventricular aneurysm.
2. Ischemic cardiomyopathy.

HOSPITAL COURSE: This was an 87-year-old lady who was visiting this area, presently to the emergency room with symptoms of acute unstable angina. She was noted to have ST-segment elevation in the inferior and anterior leads. She was brought urgently to the cardiac catheterization lab where angiography revealed total occlusion of the mid left anterior descending artery, which appeared to be an old occlusion. The right coronary artery had a 99% proximal stenosis. The left ventriculogram revealed several anteroapical hypokinesia with an aneurysm of the apex of the left ventricle. Since she was having ongoing pain, she underwent PTCA and stenting of the left coronary artery. A 3.0 x 33 cm Cypher stent was deployed with a good result. The patient did very well subsequently. However, on the date of her demise at around 12:30, the patient collapsed on her bed. She was noted to initially be in ventricular fibrillation. She was defibrillated, then she went into pulseless electrical activity despite CPR for a prolonged period time. She could not be resuscitated and was pronounced dead.

Annotations (left margin):

- s/b *presented,* incorrect term
- s/b *severe,* incorrect term
- s/b *3.0 x 33-mm,* insert hyphen, AAMT Book of Style, compound modifiers, hyphens, numbers
- s/b *mm, cm* does not make sense in a coronary vessel

Annotations (right margin):

- alt.: *DIAGNOSES,* plural
- s/b *right,* refer to body of report
- alt.: begin new paragraph to separate narrative blocks, AAMT Book of Style, formats

For Signature

DEATH SUMMARY

CLINICAL RESUME

FINAL DIAGNOSES:
1. Status post acute anterior wall myocardial infarction with left ventricular aneurysm.
2. Ischemic cardiomyopathy.

HOSPITAL COURSE: This was an 87-year-old lady who was visiting this area, presented to the emergency room with symptoms of acute unstable angina. She was noted to have ST-segment elevation in the inferior and anterior leads. She was brought urgently to the cardiac catheterization lab where angiography revealed total occlusion of the mid left anterior descending artery, which appeared to be an old occlusion. The right coronary artery had a 99% proximal stenosis. The left ventriculogram revealed severe anteroapical hypokinesia with an aneurysm of the apex of the left ventricle. Since she was having ongoing pain, she underwent PTCA and stenting of the right coronary artery. A 3.0 x 33-mm Cypher stent was deployed with a good result. The patient did very well subsequently.

However, on the date of her demise at around 12:30, the patient collapsed on her bed. She was noted to initially be in ventricular fibrillation. She was defibrillated, then she went into pulseless electrical activity despite CPR for a prolonged period time. She could not be resuscitated and was pronounced dead.

Answer Key

PSEUDOANEURYSM THROMBIN INJECTION

CARDIOVASCULAR PROCEDURE REPORT

PROCEDURE: Right groin thrombin injection under ultrasound guidance.

separate into two headings, AAMT Book of Style, formats

PREPROCEDURE AND POSTPROCEDURE DIAGNOSIS: Right groin pseudoaneurysm.

INDICATION: This is a 72-year-old female with a significant past medical history of a right groin pseudoaneurysm after a heart catheterization.

FINDINGS: She has a right groin pseudoaneurysm that was successfully thrombosed.

alt.: begin new paragraph to separate narrative blocks, AAMT Book of Style, formats

PROCEDURE: After informed written consent was obtained, the patient was placed in a supine position. The right groin was prepped and draped and, using a spinal needle, a direct thrombin injection was performed using 3000-4000 units of thrombin into the pseudoaneurysm. This abruptly occluded the pseudoaneurysm. The patient tolerated the procedure well. The patient was sent to recovery area in good condition. There were no complications.

insert *the*

For Signature

PSEUDOANEURYSM THROMBIN INJECTION

CARDIOVASCULAR PROCEDURE REPORT

PROCEDURE: Right groin thrombin injection under ultrasound guidance.

PREPROCEDURE DIAGNOSIS: Right groin pseudoaneurysm.

POSTPROCEDURE DIAGNOSIS: Right groin pseudoaneurysm.

INDICATION: This is a 72-year-old female with a significant past medical history of a right groin pseudoaneurysm after a heart catheterization.

FINDINGS: She has a right groin pseudoaneurysm that was successfully thrombosed.

PROCEDURE: After informed written consent was obtained, the patient was placed in a supine position. The right groin was prepped and draped and, using a spinal needle, a direct thrombin injection was performed using 3000-4000 units of thrombin into the pseudoaneurysm. This abruptly occluded the pseudoaneurysm.

The patient tolerated the procedure well. The patient was sent to the recovery area in good condition. There were no complications.

Answer Key

HISTORY AND PHYSICAL EXAMINATION FOR CHEST PAIN

HISTORY AND PHYSICAL EXAMINATION

CHIEF COMPLAINT: Chest pain.

HISTORY OF PRESENT ILLNESS: The patient is a 47-year-old female with a history of hypertension, gastroesophageal reflux disease, who presented to the emergency room with complaints of intermittent mid-sternal chest pain that has been ongoing for the past 3 weeks. Patient reports that her pain was worse this morning, with radiation to her back and associated shortness of breath. Patient also has a history of hypertension and has been off her medications for the past 2 weeks. She denies any associated dyspnea on exertion, fever, chills, weakness, palpitations, diaphoresis, cough, nausea, vomiting, orthopnea, congestion, or any other systems at this time. Electrocardiogram revealed normal sinus rhythm. Initial troponin was noted to be 0.01.

PAST MEDICAL HISTORY: Hypertension, gastroesophageal reflux disease, iron deficiency anemia secondary to menorrhagia.

PAST SURGICAL HISTORY: Bilateral tubal ligation.

SOCIAL HISTORY: Patient denies any alcohol, tobacco, or illicit drug use.

FAMILY HISTORY: Noncontributory.

REVIEW OF SYSTEMS: General: Patient denies fever, chills, weight loss, or weakness. Cardiovascular/respiratory: As noted in HPI. GI: Denies nausea, vomiting, diarrhea, abdominal pain, GI bleed. Neurologic: Denies headache, loss of consciousness, syncope, near syncope. Musculoskeletal: Denies joint swelling, neck pain, back pain. Eyes: Denies visual changes or pain. ENT: Denies sore throat, earache, hearing changes. Hematology: Patient has a history of iron deficiency anemia secondary to menorrhagia. Dermatology: Denies rash, pruritis, laceration, or contusion. Psychiatric: Denies depression, anxiety, suicidal or homicidal delusion or ideation. GU: Positive for urinary frequency. Denies dysuria or hematuria, vaginal discharge or bleed. Endocrine: Denies heat or cold intolerance, thyroid trouble.

(continued)

Margin notes:

s/b *midsternal*, most prefixes are joined directly to the root word, AAMT Book of Style, prefixes

s/b *symptoms*, incorrect term

s/b *near-syncope*, insert hyphen, AAMT Book of Style, compound words

s/b *Respiratory*, use initial cap for both terms when two subheadings are combined

s/b *pruritus*, misspelled, Stedman's Medical Dictionary, 28E

PHYSICAL EXAMINATION: VITAL SIGNS: Blood pressure 211/105, respirations 20, pulse 65, temperature 98.4. GENERAL: A well-developed, well-nourished 47-year-old female in no acute distress. HEENT: Normocephalic, without lesions. Sclerae, conjunctivae clear. Extraocular movements are intact. Pupils equal and reactive to light. Oropharynx within normal limits. NECK: Supple, with full range of motion. No lymphadenopathy, JVD, or bruits noted. CARDIAC: Normal S1, S2 without murmurs, gallops, or clicks present. LUNGS: Respirations even and unlabored. Lung fields without wheezes, rales, or rhonchi. CHEST: Mid-sternal epigastric tenderness noted on presentation. ABDOMEN: Soft with mild epigastric tenderness. Bowel sounds present. Liver, spleen, and kidneys not palpable. GENITOURINARY: Deferred. PELVIC/RECTAL: Deferred. EXTREMITIES: Symmetrical, without cyanosis, clubbing, edema, or varicosities. Normal range of motion of extremities noted. NEUROLOGIC: Cranial nerves 2 through 12 grossly intact. No sensory or motor deficit. INTEGUMENTARY: No open areas or lesions noted. MENTAL STATUS: Alert and oriented x3. Normal mood and affect.

LABORATORY/DIAGNOSTIC DATA: Sodium 140, potassium 3.8, chloride 110, CO2 27, BUN 12, creatinine 0.7, glucose 83. Hemoglobin 9.3, hematocrit 28.4%, platelets 303,000, WBCs 6900. Troponin 0.01, CK 216. UTI screen positive.

IMPRESSION:
1. Chest pain.
2. Accelerated hypertension.
3. Gastroesophageal reflux disease.
4. History of iron deficiency anemia secondary to menorrhagia.
5. Urinary frequency.
6. Rule out urinary tract infection.
7. Medication noncompliance.

s/b Midsternal

NOTE: arabic numbers are acceptable, AAMT Book of Style, numbers, cranial nerves

For Signature

HISTORY AND PHYSICAL EXAMINATION FOR CHEST PAIN

HISTORY AND PHYSICAL EXAMINATION

CHIEF COMPLAINT: Chest pain.

HISTORY OF PRESENT ILLNESS: The patient is a 47-year-old female with a history of hypertension, gastroesophageal reflux disease, who presented to the emergency room with complaints of intermittent midsternal chest pain that has been ongoing for the past three weeks. Patient reports that her pain was worse this morning, with radiation to her back and associated shortness of breath. Patient also has a history of hypertension and has been off her medications for the past two weeks. She denies any associated dyspnea on exertion, fever, chills, weakness, palpitations, diaphoresis, cough, nausea, vomiting, orthopnea, congestion, or any other symptoms at this time. Electrocardiogram revealed normal sinus rhythm. Initial troponin was noted to be 0.01.

PAST MEDICAL HISTORY: Hypertension, gastroesophageal reflux disease, iron deficiency anemia secondary to menorrhagia.

PAST SURGICAL HISTORY: Bilateral tubal ligation.

SOCIAL HISTORY: Patient denies any alcohol, tobacco, or illicit drug use.

FAMILY HISTORY: Noncontributory.

REVIEW OF SYSTEMS: General: Patient denies fever, chills, weight loss or weakness. Cardiovascular/Respiratory: As noted in HPI. GI: Denies nausea, vomiting, diarrhea, abdominal pain, GI bleed. Neurologic: Denies headache, loss of consciousness, syncope, near-syncope. Musculoskeletal: Denies joint swelling, neck pain, back pain. Eyes: Denies visual changes or pain. ENT: Denies sore throat, earache, hearing changes. Hematology: Patient has a history of iron deficiency anemia secondary to menorrhagia. Dermatology: Denies rash, pruritus, laceration, or contusion. Psychiatric: Denies depression, anxiety, suicidal or homicidal delusion or ideation. GU: Positive for urinary frequency. Denies dysuria or hematuria, vaginal discharge or bleed. Endocrine: Denies heat or cold intolerance, thyroid trouble.

PHYSICAL EXAMINATION: VITAL SIGNS: Blood pressure 211/105, respirations 20, pulse 65, temperature 98.4. GENERAL: A well-developed, well-nourished 47-year-old female in no acute distress. HEENT: Normocephalic, without lesions. Sclerae, conjunctivae clear. Extraocular movements are intact. Pupils equal and reactive to light. Oropharynx within normal limits. NECK: Supple, with full range of motion. No lymphadenopathy, JVD, or bruits noted. CARDIAC: Normal S1, S2 without murmurs, gallops, or clicks present. LUNGS: Respirations even and unlabored. Lung fields without wheezes, rales, or rhonchi. CHEST: Midsternal epigastric tenderness noted on presentation. ABDOMEN: Soft with mild epigastric tenderness. Bowel sounds present. Liver, spleen, and kidneys not palpable. GENITOURINARY: Deferred. PELVIC/RECTAL: Deferred. EXTREMITIES: Symmetrical, without cyanosis, clubbing, edema, or varicosities. Normal range of

(continued)

motion of extremities noted. NEUROLOGIC: Cranial nerves 2 through 12 grossly intact. No sensory or motor deficit. INTEGUMENTARY: No open areas or lesions noted. MENTAL STATUS: Alert and oriented x3. Normal mood and affect.

LABORATORY/DIAGNOSTIC DATA: Sodium 140, potassium 3.8, chloride 110, CO_2 27, BUN 12, creatinine 0.7, glucose 83. Hemoglobin 9.3, hematocrit 28.4%, platelets 303,000, WBCs 6900. Troponin 0.01, CK 216. UTI screen positive.

IMPRESSION:
1. Chest pain.
2. Accelerated hypertension.
3. Gastroesophageal reflux disease.
4. History of iron deficiency anemia secondary to menorrhagia.
5. Urinary frequency.
6. Rule out urinary tract infection.
7. Medication noncompliance.

Answer Key

Report #5

ABDOMINAL AORTOGRAM WITH LOWER EXTREMITY RUNOFF

CARDIAC IMAGING

PROCEDURE PERFORMED: Abdominal aortogram with lower extremity runoff.

CLINICAL HISTORY: The patient is a 66-year-old female with a history of intermittent claudication, as well as a family history of aneurysms. She comes in today for evaluation.

DESCRIPTION: The patient was brought to the catheterization laboratory in a stable, fasting condition. The right groin was prepped and draped in the usual fashion. A 5-French sheath was placed without difficulty in the left femoral artery using modified Seldinger technique. A 5-French marker pigtail catheter was placed in the abdominal aorta. Abdominal aortography was performed with the catheter placed just above the renal artery takeoff. The catheter was then brought down to just above the aortoiliac junction, and digitally subtracted lower extremity angiography was performed bilaterally. Sheath was sewn in to be removed later in the postcatheterization area, after the catheter was removed over a wire. The patient tolerated the procedure without any problems in the laboratory. Contrast, total of 80 cc, was used.

FINDINGS:

ABDOMINAL AORTOGRAM: Smooth and free of significant disease.

LOWER EXTREMITIES RUNOFF:

Right lower extremity: The vessels were all seen pretty well and appeared to be free of significant plaque or ectasia.

Left lower extremity: The vessels of the left leg showed some minimal plaquing with maximal stenosis of 40% seen in the proximal common femoral artery.

IMPRESSION:

Pretty normal study. No evidence of significant occlusive disease.

RECOMMENDATIONS:

Reassurance.

Margin annotations:

insert hyphen to connect adjectival phrase describing a noun, AAMT Book of Style, hyphens

alt.: for clarity change to: *A total of 80 mL of contrast was used.*

s/b *EXTREMITY*, singular

move to same line as heading for format continuity

it is unclear as to whether this should be the left or the right femoral artery; flag the report to follow up with the physician, AAMT Book of Style, dictation problems

alt.: recast for clarity to: *The catheter was removed over a wire. The sheath was sewn in, to be removed later in the post-catheterization area.*

s/b *mL*, ISMP List of Dangerous Abbreviations

alt.: delete redundant words

For Signature

Report #5

ABDOMINAL AORTOGRAM WITH LOWER EXTREMITY RUNOFF

FLAG: Doctor, please clarify whether it should be the left or the right femoral artery under DESCRIPTION, 3rd line down. Thank you.

CARDIAC IMAGING

PROCEDURE PERFORMED: Abdominal aortogram with lower extremity runoff.

CLINICAL HISTORY: The patient is a 66-year-old female with a history of intermittent claudication, as well as a family history of aneurysms. She comes in today for evaluation.

DESCRIPTION: The patient was brought to the catheterization laboratory in a stable, fasting condition. The right groin was prepped and draped in the usual fashion. A 5-French sheath was placed without difficulty in the <u>left femoral artery</u> using modified Seldinger technique. A 5-French marker pigtail catheter was placed in the abdominal aorta. Abdominal aortography was performed with the catheter placed just above the renal artery takeoff. The catheter was then brought down to just above the aortoiliac junction, and digitally subtracted lower extremity angiography was performed bilaterally. The catheter was removed over a wire. The sheath was sewn in, to be removed later in the postcatheterization area. The patient tolerated the procedure without any problems in the laboratory. A total of 80 mL of contrast was used.

FINDINGS:

ABDOMINAL AORTOGRAM: Smooth and free of significant disease.

LOWER EXTREMITY RUNOFF:

Right lower extremity: The vessels were all seen well and appeared to be free of significant plaque or ectasia.

Left lower extremity: The vessels of the left leg showed minimal plaquing with maximal stenosis of 40% seen in the proximal common femoral artery.

IMPRESSION: Normal study with no evidence of significant occlusive disease.

RECOMMENDATIONS: Reassurance.

Answer Key

Report #6

M-MODE, TWO-DIMENSIONAL AND DOPPLER ECHOCARDIOGRAM

CARDIOLOGY PROCEDURE REPORT

PROCEDURE: Echocardiogram.

REFERRING PHYSICIAN: XXXX

CLINICAL INDICATIONS: Syncope.

TYPE OF PROCEDURE: M-mode, 2-D and Doppler echocardiogram.

DESCRIPTION:

M-MODE AND TWO-DIMENSIONAL FINDINGS: Technically fair study done in standard, multiple views. Grossly, all four cardiac chambers have normal dimensions. The left ventricular systolic function is normal. Regional wall motion abnormalities are not detracted. Mild concentric left ventricular hypertrophy is noted; left ventricular ejection fraction is approximately 6%. Mitral, tricuspid and aortic valves appear to be grossly normal except for minimal calcification. Right-sided chambers are normal. Pericardial effusion is absent. No thrombi is seen in the left ventricle.

DOPPLER REPORT: Doppler echocardiographic analysis reveals trace mitral, tricuspid and aortic regurgitation. There is evidence of repaired relaxation of the left ventricle, consistent with diastolic dysfunction.

CONCLUSION:
1. Left ventricular systolic function is normal with an ejection fraction estimated to be approximately 6%.
2. Regional wall motion abnormalities are absent.
3. No significant valvular abnormalities are present.
4. Pericardial effusion is absent.
5. Intracardiac mass or thrombus is absent.

s/b detected, incorrect term

s/b either thrombus is or thrombi are, subject/verb agreement

s/b impaired, incorrect term

s/b 60%, typographical error; an ejection fraction of 6% does not make sense in the context of normal left ventricular systolic function, Stedman's Medical Dictionary, 28E, ejection fraction

For Signature

Report #6

M-MODE, TWO-DIMENSIONAL AND DOPPLER ECHOCARDIOGRAM

CARDIOLOGY PROCEDURE REPORT

PROCEDURE: Echocardiogram.

REFERRING PHYSICIAN: XXXX

CLINICAL INDICATIONS: Syncope.

TYPE OF PROCEDURE: M-mode, 2-D and Doppler echocardiogram.

DESCRIPTION:

M-MODE AND TWO-DIMENSIONAL FINDINGS: Technically fair study done in standard, multiple views. Grossly, all four cardiac chambers have normal dimensions. The left ventricular systolic function is normal. Regional wall motion abnormalities are not detected. Mild concentric left ventricular hypertrophy is noted; left ventricular ejection fraction is approximately 60%. Mitral, tricuspid and aortic valves appear to be grossly normal except for minimal calcification. Right-sided chambers are normal. Pericardial effusion is absent. No thrombus is seen in the left ventricle.

DOPPLER REPORT: Doppler echocardiographic analysis reveals trace mitral, tricuspid and aortic regurgitation. There is evidence of impaired relaxation of the left ventricle, consistent with diastolic dysfunction.

CONCLUSION:
1. Left ventricular systolic function is normal with an ejection fraction estimated to be approximately 60%.
2. Regional wall motion abnormalities are absent.
3. No significant valvular abnormalities are present.
4. Pericardial effusion is absent.
5. Intracardiac mass or thrombus is absent.

Answer Key

HOLTER MONITOR

HOLTER MONITOR REPORT

PROCEDURE TYPE: A 24-hour Holter monitor.

INDICATIONS: A 74-year-old female complaining of "heart fluttering." Test is being done to evaluate.

FINDINGS:
1. Basic rhythm is sinus rhythm.
2. Average heart rate of 72 beats per minute, minimum heart rate 54 beats per minute, maximum heart rate 98 beats per minute at peak.
3. Competent PR interval, QRS, ST within normal limits.
4. Rare ventricular ectopic beats were seen; total number of ventricular ectopic beats in 24 hours were 6. There were no couplets, triplets, or runs of nonsustained or sustained ventricular tachycardia.
5. Rare atrial ectopic beats were seen; total number of atrial ectopic beats in 24 hours were 7. There were no runs of ventricular tachycardia.
6. No significant bradyarrhythmias seen.
7. Patient did not report any symptoms in the diary.

CONCLUSION:
1. Basic rhythm is sinus.
2. Rare atrial ectopic beats without runs of atrial tachycardia.
3. Rare ventricular ectopic beats without couplets, triplets, or runs of nonsustained or sustained ventricular tachycardia.
4. Patient did not report any symptoms in the diary.

alt.: delete *of*, unnecessary

replace comma with a semicolon for clarity

s/b *was*, incorrect tense; verb refers to *number* (singular), not to *beats* (plural)

For Signature

HOLTER MONITOR

HOLTER MONITOR REPORT

PROCEDURE TYPE: A 24-hour Holter monitor.

INDICATIONS: A 74-year-old female complaining of "heart fluttering." Test is being done to evaluate.

FINDINGS:
1. Basic rhythm is sinus rhythm.
2. Average heart rate 72 beats per minute, minimum heart rate 54 beats per minute, maximum heart rate 98 beats per minute at peak.
3. Competent PR interval; QRS, ST within normal limits.
4. Rare ventricular ectopic beats were seen; total number of ventricular ectopic beats in 24 hours was 6. There were no couplets, triplets, or runs of nonsustained or sustained ventricular tachycardia.
5. Rare atrial ectopic beats were seen; total number of atrial ectopic beats in 24 hours was 7. There were no runs of ventricular tachycardia.
6. No significant bradyarrhythmias seen.
7. Patient did not report any symptoms in the diary.

CONCLUSION:
1. Basic rhythm is sinus.
2. Rare atrial ectopic beats without runs of atrial tachycardia.
3. Rare ventricular ectopic beats without couplets, triplets, or runs of nonsustained or sustained ventricular tachycardia.
4. Patient did not report any symptoms in the diary.

Answer Key

THORACIC ARCH ARTERIOGRAPHY TO VISUALIZE CAROTID ARTERIES

In cardiology, arteriography and angiography are used synonymously. In this report, the originator refers to aortography during the descriptive portion of the dictation. This is not said in error, as the aorta would have to be imaged in order to do a thoracic arch study.

VASCULAR IMAGING

PROCEDURES:

1. Thoracic arch arteriography.
2. Selective carotid arteriography.

PREPROCEDURE DIAGNOSIS:

Right carotid artery stenosis.

POSTPROCEDURE DIAGNOSIS:

Right carotid artery stenosis.

SUMMARY OF RADIOGRAPHIC FINDINGS:

Right carotid stenosis, 80%. Patent anterior and middle cerebral arteries. No intracoronary pathology. Easily cannulated common carotid artery with a Simmons 2.

> *s/b intracerebral, incorrect term*

> *s/b weekly, misspelled*

INDICATIONS: This is a 71-year-old gentleman with renal insufficiency, COPD, coronary artery disease, CABG surgeries in 1983 and 1984, PTCA, CVA, and pacemaker, with episodic weakly stable angina and chest pain. He has an asymptomatic carotid artery stenosis.

> *delete an*

TECHNIQUE:

> *move below heading for format continuity*

After informed written consent was obtained, the patient was taken to the catheterization laboratory, placed in the supine position. After intravenous sedation was administered, the patient was prepped and draped in the usual sterile fashion. Via modified Seldinger technique, a direct puncture was made into the left common carotid artery. Wires and catheters were inserted to the level of the thoracic arch. A 5-French sheath was inserted with a pigtail catheter. Aortography was performed. A Simmons 2 catheter was used to cannulate the carotid arteries, and carotid angiography was performed. Upon termination of the procedure, all wires and catheters were removed. Patient tolerated the

> *alt.: delete comma, insert and for clarity*

(continued)

procedure well. The patient was sent to the recovery area in good condition.

FINDINGS:

The right internal carotid artery shows a carotid artery stenosis of approximately 80% to 90%, with involvement of the bifurcation; that is, it is not above or below the bifurcation. This is a very straight internal carotid artery. There is a normal arch configuration. All intracerebral vessels are observed. There is no intracerebral pathology.

FINAL IMPRESSION:

Right coronary artery stenosis, 80%.

s/b carotid,
incorrect term

For Signature

THORACIC ARCH ARTERIOGRAPHY TO VISUALIZE CAROTID ARTERIES

VASCULAR IMAGING

PROCEDURES:

1. Thoracic arch arteriography.
2. Selective carotid arteriography.

PREPROCEDURE DIAGNOSIS:

Right carotid artery stenosis.

POSTPROCEDURE DIAGNOSIS:

Right carotid artery stenosis.

SUMMARY OF RADIOGRAPHIC FINDINGS:

Right carotid stenosis, 80%. Patent anterior and middle cerebral arteries. No intracerebral pathology. Easily cannulated common carotid artery with a Simmons 2.

INDICATIONS:

This is a 71-year-old gentleman with renal insufficiency, COPD, coronary artery disease, CABG surgeries in 1983 and 1984, PTCA, CVA, and pacemaker, with episodic weekly stable angina and chest pain. He has asymptomatic carotid artery stenosis.

TECHNIQUE:

After informed written consent was obtained, the patient was taken to the catheterization laboratory and placed in the supine position. After intravenous sedation was administered, the patient was prepped and draped in the usual sterile fashion. Via modified Seldinger technique, a direct puncture was made into the left common carotid artery. Wires and catheters were inserted to the level of the thoracic arch. A 5-French sheath was inserted with a pigtail catheter. Aortography was performed. A Simmons 2 catheter was used to cannulate the carotid arteries, and carotid angiography was performed. Upon termination of the procedure, all wires and catheters were removed. Patient tolerated the procedure well. The patient was sent to the recovery area in good condition.

FINDINGS:

The right internal carotid artery shows a carotid artery stenosis of approximately 80% to 90%, with involvement of the bifurcation; that is, it is not above or below the bifurcation. This is a very straight internal carotid artery. There is a normal arch configuration. All intracerebral vessels are observed. There is no intracerebral pathology.

FINAL IMPRESSION:

Right carotid artery stenosis, 80%.

Answer Key   Report #9

HISTORY AND PHYSICAL EXAMINATION

CHIEF COMPLAINT/HISTORY OF PRESENT ILLNESS: Patient is a 78-year-old male who came to the emergency room this morning with shortness of breath. He stated that this started about two days ago when he had sharp, crampy pains across the lower chest that were quite severe. The next night, that is last night, he was severely short of breath, but it gradually started subsiding. The pains did not recur. This morning he awoke and again had severe shortness of breath, thus came to the emergency room for evaluation. No more chest pains have been reported. He describes no leg pain, however, there has been some slight swelling in the legs, particularly the left leg. He does have some mild, chronic leg cramping and swelling.

> change comma to semicolon, AAMT Book of Style, however

PAST MEDICAL HISTORY: Pertinent for a ventricular septal defect with secondary pulmonary hypertension. He also has hypertensive cardiovascular disease. The patient is obese. He also has a history of a nonischemic cardiomyopathy, probably related to the VSD, as well as a history of renal insufficiency, hyperlipidemia and AR.

PAST SURGICAL HISTORY: Previous surgeries as per old records.

ALLERGIES: NO KNOWN ALLERGIES TO MEDICATIONS.

> NOTE: AAMT Book of Style, allergies, states: "Some institutions use capitals or bold type to draw attention to a patient's allergies. Regular type is, of course, also acceptable. Do not underline or use italics; either reduces readability."

MEDICATIONS: Routine medications currently include Singular 10 mg daily, Pravachol 20 mg daily, Toprol XL 50 mg daily, fosinopril 40 mg daily, Norvasc 5 mg daily, Plavix 7.5 mg daily, Clarinex 5 mg daily, spironolactone 25 mg daily, Lasix 40 mg daily.

> s/b *Toprol-XL*, Quick Look Drug Book 2006

> s/b 75, incorrect dosage, Quick Look Drug Book 2006

SOCIAL HISTORY: Nonsmoker, nondrinker.

FAMILY HISTORY: Noncontributory.

REVIEW OF SYSTEMS: Essentially as above. Denies fevers or chills. Denies head or chest cold symptoms. Denies any worsening of his allergies or baseline breathing problems, except for above. No stomach pains or cramps, nausea or vomiting. Bowels have been moving regularly. No visible blood in the stool or urine. No burning or pain on urination.

(continued)

PHYSICAL EXAMINATION:

GENERAL: Obese white male in no acute distress.

VITAL SIGNS: Vital signs in the emergency room included a blood pressure of 143/89, respirations 20, pulse 130 and regular, temperature 98.4, O2 saturation 95% on room air.

HEENT: EOMs full. Pupils reactive. Mucus membranes minimally dry.

s/b mucous, misspelled, Stedman's Medical Dictionary, 28E

NECK: Supple, no adenopathy, no thyromegaly, no appreciable bruits in the neck.

CHEST: No adenopathy.

LUNGS: Lung fields revealed bibasilar crackles, more so on the left.

HEART: Regular; a harsh systolic murmur at the left upper sternal border. PMI was displaced bilaterally.

s/b laterally, incorrect term

ABDOMEN: Soft, bowel sounds were active. No organomegaly. No masses, guarding or rebound.

RECTAL: Rectal referred to office.

s/b deferred, incorrect term

EXTREMITIES: Full range of motion. Lower extremities had 2+ pedal edema, left greater than right, with bilateral venous stasis changes.

NEUROLOGIC: Grossly intact, without focal deficits.

DATA: Laboratory data include initial negative cardiac enzymes. D-dimer was 6.6. BMP was 562. Initial chemistries with a creatinine of 1.9, potassium 4.5, LFTs unremarkable, CBC was unremarkable, including a normal white cell count. A CT scan of the chest was reported, unofficially, as showing changes at both bases, consistent with pulmonary emboli.

s/b BNP (brain or b naturetic peptid); BMP is a panel of several labs and would not have only one numeric value listed

IMPRESSION:
1. Probable bilateral basilar pulmonary emboli.
2. Shortness of breath, suspect secondary to above, however, cannot exclude acute decompensated heart failure.
3. History of ventricular septal defect with secondary pulmonary hypertension.
4. Nonischemic cardiomyopathy with prior history of congestive heart failure.
5. Obesity.
6. Renal insufficiency.
7. Hypertensive cardiovascular disease.
8. Hyperlipidemia.
9. Aortic regurgitation.

change comma to semicolon, AAMT Book of Style, however

(continued)

ANSWER KEYS AND FOR SIGNATURE REPORTS

s/b *Pulmonary*, capitalize a department name that is referred to as an entity, AAMT Book of Style, business names, departments

insert blank line for format continuity

PLAN: At this time, patient will be admitted for further evaluation and therapy. He will be started immediately on heparin. Cardiology and pulmonary will be consulted. He will be kept on bed rest. Will continue his usual medications except for the Plavix. Monitor hemoglobin.
Patient may eventually require a Greenfield filter. Further treatment depends upon clinical course and findings.

For Signature

HISTORY AND PHYSICAL EXAMINATION FOR SHORTNESS OF BREATH

HISTORY AND PHYSICAL EXAMINATION

CHIEF COMPLAINT/HISTORY OF PRESENT ILLNESS: Patient is a 78-year-old male who came to the emergency room this morning with shortness of breath. He stated that this started about two days ago when he had sharp, crampy pains across the lower chest that were quite severe. The next night, that is last night, he was severely short of breath, but it gradually started subsiding. The pains did not recur. This morning he awoke and again had severe shortness of breath, thus came to the emergency room for evaluation. No more chest pains have been reported. He describes no leg pain; however, there has been some slight swelling in the legs, particularly the left leg. He does have some mild, chronic leg cramping and swelling.

PAST MEDICAL HISTORY: Pertinent for a ventricular septal defect with secondary pulmonary hypertension. He also has hypertensive cardiovascular disease. The patient is obese. He also has a history of a nonischemic cardiomyopathy, probably related to the VSD, as well as a history of renal insufficiency, hyperlipidemia and AR.

PAST SURGICAL HISTORY: Previous surgeries as per old records.

ALLERGIES: NO KNOWN ALLERGIES TO MEDICATIONS.

MEDICATIONS: Routine medications currently include Singular 10 mg daily, Pravachol 20 mg daily, Toprol-XL 50 mg daily, fosinopril 40 mg daily, Norvasc 5 mg daily, Plavix 75 mg daily, Clarinex 5 mg daily, spironolactone 25 mg daily, Lasix 40 mg daily.

SOCIAL HISTORY: Nonsmoker, nondrinker.

FAMILY HISTORY: Noncontributory.

REVIEW OF SYSTEMS: Essentially as above. Denies fevers or chills. Denies head or chest cold symptoms. Denies any worsening of his allergies or baseline breathing problems, except for above. No stomach pains or cramps, nausea or vomiting. Bowels have been moving regularly. No visible blood in the stool or urine. No burning or pain on urination.

PHYSICAL EXAMINATION:

GENERAL: Obese white male in no acute distress.

VITAL SIGNS: Vital signs in the emergency room included a blood pressure of 143/89, respirations 20, pulse 130 and regular, temperature 98.4, O2 saturation 95% on room air.

HEENT: EOMs full. Pupils reactive. Mucous membranes minimally dry.

NECK: Supple, no adenopathy, no thyromegaly, no appreciable bruits in the neck.

CHEST: No adenopathy.

(continued)

LUNGS: Lung fields revealed bibasilar crackles, more so on the left.

HEART: Regular; a harsh systolic murmur at the left upper sternal border. PMI was displaced laterally.

ABDOMEN: Soft, bowel sounds were active. No organomegaly. No masses, guarding or rebound.

RECTAL: Rectal deferred to office.

EXTREMITIES: Full range of motion. Lower extremities had 2+ pedal edema, left greater than right, with bilateral venous stasis changes.

NEUROLOGIC: Grossly intact, without focal deficits.

DATA: Laboratory data include initial negative cardiac enzymes. D-dimer was 6.6. BNP was 562. Initial chemistries with a creatinine of 1.9, potassium 4.5, LFTs unremarkable, CBC was unremarkable, including a normal white cell count. A CT scan of the chest was reported, unofficially, as showing changes at both bases, consistent with pulmonary emboli.

IMPRESSION:
1. Probable bilateral basilar pulmonary emboli.
2. Shortness of breath, suspect secondary to above; however, cannot exclude acute decompensated heart failure.
3. History of ventricular septal defect with secondary pulmonary hypertension.
4. Nonischemic cardiomyopathy with prior history of congestive heart failure.
5. Obesity.
6. Renal insufficiency.
7. Hypertensive cardiovascular disease.
8. Hyperlipidemia.
9. Aortic regurgitation.

PLAN: At this time, patient will be admitted for further evaluation and therapy. He will be started immediately on heparin. Cardiology and Pulmonary will be consulted. He will be kept on bed rest. Will continue his usual medications except for the Plavix. Monitor hemoglobin.

Patient may eventually require a Greenfield filter. Further treatment depends upon clinical course and findings.

Answer Key

INFERIOR VENA CAVA FILTER PLACEMENT FOR PATIENT CONTRAINDICATED FOR ANTICOAGULATION

VASCULAR INTERVENTION PROCEDURE

PROCEDURE PERFORMED: Inferior vena cava filter placement.

PREPROCEDURE DIAGNOSIS: Pulmonary embolism.

POSTPROCEDURE DIAGNOSIS: Pulmonary embolism.

SURGEON: XXXX

INDICATIONS: Pulmonary embolism with DVT and bleeding; contraindication to anticoagulation.

ESTIMATED BLOOD LOSS: Minimal. No blood products given.

COUNTS: All counts were correct.

ACCESS: Right internal jugular vein.

SYSTEM: Trapeze.

s/b TrapEase, incorrect spelling, Stedman's Cardiovascular & Pulmonary Words, 4E

PROCEDURE: After informed written consent was obtained, the patient was taken to the OR and placed in supine position. Intravenous sedation was administered. The patient was prepped and draped in the usual sterile fashion. After an appropriate amount of local anesthesia was given over the right internal jugular vein, a direct puncture was made into the vessel, and wires and catheters were inserted up into the inferior vena cava. An inferior venacavagram was performed and IVC filter was put below the renal veins. The patient tolerated the procedure well. There were no complications.

s/b down; anatomically, going from the internal jugular vein to the inferior vena cava signifies down

SUMMARY OF RADIOGRAPHIC FINDINGS:
1. Patient IVC.
2. Normal deployment of an inferior vena cava filter.

s/b patent, incorrect word

DISPOSITION: An IVC filter was placed just below the renal veins, in good position. There were no complications.

For Signature

INFERIOR VENA CAVA FILTER PLACEMENT FOR PATIENT CONTRAINDICATED FOR ANTICOAGULATION

VASCULAR INTERVENTION PROCEDURE

PROCEDURE PERFORMED: Inferior vena cava filter placement.

PREPROCEDURE DIAGNOSIS: Pulmonary embolism.

POSTPROCEDURE DIAGNOSIS: Pulmonary embolism.

SURGEON: XXXX

INDICATIONS: Pulmonary embolism with DVT and bleeding; contraindication to anticoagulation.

ESTIMATED BLOOD LOSS: Minimal. No blood products given.

COUNTS: All counts were correct.

ACCESS: Right internal jugular vein.

SYSTEM: TrapEase.

PROCEDURE: After informed written consent was obtained, the patient was taken to the OR and placed in supine position. Intravenous sedation was administered. The patient was prepped and draped in the usual sterile fashion. After an appropriate amount of local anesthesia was given over the right internal jugular vein, a direct puncture was made into the vessel and wires and catheters were inserted down into the inferior vena cava. An inferior venacavagram was performed and IVC filter was put below the renal veins. The patient tolerated the procedure well. There were no complications.

SUMMARY OF RADIOGRAPHIC FINDINGS:
1. Patent IVC.
2. Normal deployment of an inferior vena cava filter.

DISPOSITION: An IVC filter was placed just below the renal veins, in good position. There were no complications.

Answer Key

HISTORY AND PHYSICAL EXAMINATION FOR ATRIAL FIBRILLATION

HISTORY AND PHYSICAL EXAMINATION

CHIEF COMPLAINT: Chest pressure, palpitations.

HISTORY OF PRESENT ILLNESS: Patient is a 72-year-old white male with a past medical history significant for hypertension, coronary artery disease; he had a CABG done in March 2005. He had atrial fibrillation just prior to this surgery. He was doing very well until this morning, when he started having the feeling of palpations, plus feeling pressure in his chest, on the left side. He came into the emergency room for further evaluation. At home, he checked his blood pressure which was in the 90s. His heart rate went from the low 40s to as high as 150. In the emergency room, he had an initial evaluation with blood work and cardiac enzymes. She is being admitted to rule out MI protocol and evaluation of his atrial fibrillation.

s/b palpitations, misspelled

s/b He

PAST MEDICAL HISTORY: Significant for coronary artery disease, hypertension, and CABG in March 2005.

MEDICATIONS: At home he takes alprazolam, Zoloft, lisinopril, Plavix, Zocor, Toprol, Nexium, aspirin, and Allegra.

SOCIAL HISTORY: Patient lives at home with his wife. Patient does not smoke or drink alcohol.

FAMILY HISTORY: Noncontributory.

REVIEW OF SYSTEMS: Patient denies any temperature, any chills, any headache, any visual changes. Denies any shortness of breath, any cough. Denies any abdominal pain or any problem with bowels or bladder.

PHYSICAL EXAMINATION:

GENERAL: Physical exam shows a pleasant white man.

VITAL SIGNS: Blood pressure 112/48, heart rate 62, temperature 98.2.

HEENT: Head: Normocephalic, atraumatic. Eyes: Pupils round, reactive to light and accommodation; extraocular muscles intact. Mouth: Moist, no lesion.

NECK: No JVD, no bruit.

(continued)

LUNGS: Clear to auscultation and percussion.

HEART: Regularly irregular. S1, S2. No murmur.

ABDOMEN: Soft; positive bowel sounds.

EXTREMITIES: No edema.

NEUROLOGIC: Patient is alert, oriented, without any focal deficit.

LABORATORY/DIAGNOSTIC DATA: His labs show sodium 137, potassium 4.1, BUN 12, creatinine 0.9. White blood count 7500, hemoglobin and hematocrit of 42.6 and 14.7. His CPK initially was 39, troponin less than 0.01. ECG did not show any acute changes. A chest x-ray was within normal limits.

IMPRESSION:
1. Chest pressure, atrial fibrillation, new onset.
2. Hypertension.
3. History of coronary artery disease.

PLAN: Will admit patient to a monitored bed for rule out MI protocol and for rhythm evaluation. Will consult his cardiologist and will continue his home medications.

s/b *hemoglobin and hematocrit of 14.7 and 42.6,* Stedman's Pathology & Lab Medicine Words, 4E, Appendix 8. NOTE: It is common for hemoglobin and hematocrit values to be transposed; familiarize yourself with the expected values for each

For Signature

HISTORY AND PHYSICAL EXAMINATION FOR ATRIAL FIBRILLATION

HISTORY AND PHYSICAL EXAMINATION

CHIEF COMPLAINT: Chest pressure, palpitations.

HISTORY OF PRESENT ILLNESS: Patient is a 72-year-old white male with a past medical history significant for hypertension, coronary artery disease; he had a CABG done in March 2005. He had atrial fibrillation just prior to this surgery. He was doing very well until this morning, when he started having the feeling of palpitations, plus feeling pressure in his chest, on the left side. He came into the emergency room for further evaluation. At home, he checked his blood pressure which was in the 90s. His heart rate went from the low 40s to as high as 150. In the emergency room, he had an initial evaluation with blood work and cardiac enzymes. He is being admitted to rule out MI protocol and evaluation of his atrial fibrillation.

PAST MEDICAL HISTORY: Significant for coronary artery disease, hypertension, and CABG in March 2005.

MEDICATIONS: At home he takes alprazolam, Zoloft, lisinopril, Plavix, Zocor, Toprol, Nexium, aspirin, and Allegra.

SOCIAL HISTORY: Patient lives at home with his wife. Patient does not smoke or drink alcohol.

FAMILY HISTORY: Noncontributory.

REVIEW OF SYSTEMS: Patient denies any temperature, any chills, any headache, any visual changes. Denies any shortness of breath, any cough. Denies any abdominal pain or any problem with bowels or bladder.

PHYSICAL EXAMINATION:

GENERAL: Physical exam shows a pleasant white man.

VITAL SIGNS: Blood pressure 112/48, heart rate 62, temperature 98.2.

HEENT: Head: Normocephalic, atraumatic. Eyes: Pupils round, reactive to light and accommodation; extraocular muscles intact. Mouth: Moist, no lesion.

NECK: No JVD, no bruit.

LUNGS: Clear to auscultation and percussion.

HEART: Regularly irregular. S1, S2. No murmur.

ABDOMEN: Soft; positive bowel sounds.

EXTREMITIES: No edema.

NEUROLOGIC: Patient is alert, oriented, without any focal deficit.

(continued)

LABORATORY/DIAGNOSTIC DATA: His labs show sodium 137, potassium 4.1, BUN 12, creatinine 0.9. White blood count 7500, hemoglobin and hematocrit of 14.7 and 42.6. His CPK initially was 39, troponin less than 0.01. ECG did not show any acute changes. A chest x-ray was within normal limits.

IMPRESSION:
1. Chest pressure, atrial fibrillation, new onset.
2. Hypertension.
3. History of coronary artery disease.

PLAN: Will admit patient to a monitored bed for rule out MI protocol and for rhythm evaluation. Will consult his cardiologist and will continue his home medications.

Answer Key

Report #12

NORMAL PERSANTINE THALLIUM STRESS TEST

Dipyridamole is the generic form of Persantine; frequently physicians refer to them both interchangeably during dictation. It is not necessary to have the same name for the medication throughout the study, though not incorrect to change the name for the sake of continuity. This would be best determined by facility/department requirements.

CARDIAC IMAGING

PROCEDURE: Persantine thallium _____ — insert period

INDICATIONS: A 70-year-old admitted with atypical chest pain.

BASELINE: Resting electrocardiogram shows sinus rhythm, normal EKG.

PERSANTINE THALLIUM: The patient received an injection of Persantine per standard protocol. The resting heart rate was 70, which decreased to 82 after dipyridamole. The resting blood pressure was 104/50, which did not change. The patient denied chest pain. No ECG changes. No arrhythmias.

s/b showed for uniformity in tense

s/b increased

s/b EKG for uniformity

CONCLUSION:
1. Normal electrocardiographic response to dipyridamole.
2. Normal hemodynamic response to dipyridamole.
3. No chest pain during the test.
4. No arrhythmias.
5. The results of the thallium portion of the test were pending at the time of the dictation.

For Signature

NORMAL PERSANTINE THALLIUM STRESS TEST

CARDIAC IMAGING

PROCEDURE: Persantine thallium.

INDICATIONS: A 70-year-old admitted with atypical chest pain.

BASELINE: Resting electrocardiogram showed sinus rhythm, normal EKG.

PERSANTINE THALLIUM: The patient received an injection of Persantine per standard protocol. The resting heart rate was 70, which increased to 82 after dipyridamole. The resting blood pressure was 104/50, which did not change. The patient denied chest pain. No EKG changes. No arrhythmias.

CONCLUSION:
1. Normal electrocardiographic response to dipyridamole.
2. Normal hemodynamic response to dipyridamole.
3. No chest pain during the test.
4. No arrhythmias.
5. The results of the thallium portion of the test were pending at the time of the dictation.

Answer Key

CONSULTATION FOR CHEST PAIN

CONSULTATION

ATTENDING: XXXX

CONSULTANT: XXXX

CHIEF COMPLAINT: Chest pain.

FINDINGS AND RECOMMENDATIONS OF CONSULTANT: The patient is a pleasant 84-year-old gentleman with multiple medical problems. He has a history of multivessel stenting, history of EF of 45% to 50%, with a recent admission for CHF, with elevated BNP, and also a urinary tract infection. According to his son, he was being transported in a van to a nursing home after a visit outside the nursing home and, in the process of transport, the patient developed chest pain. It may be musculoskeletal in nature, but the patient describes some heaviness associated with palpitations. He does have a history of coronary disease and has numerous other medical problems as well. He is a fairly poor historian, and most of the information obtained is form the patient's son. In terms of the ECG, he has evidence of T wave inversions seen in I and aVL. His first set of enzymes are pending. The patient also has severe peripheral vascular disease, has a history of chronic constipation, has a history of renal insufficiency, multiple myeloma as well and has had a history of a left lower extremity DVT leading to being placed on chronic anticoagulation. He also has a history of anemia and has had prior GI workup, the records of which are unavailable at this time. Patient describes some reproducible chest pain with palpation, but no diaphoresis and no radiation of the pain to the back; no orthopnea or PND.

REVIEW OF SYSTEMS: General: No fevers, chills, weight loss or weakness. Cardiovascular: See the HPI. Respiratory: See the HPI. GI: No nausea, vomiting, diarrhea; no abdominal pain or GI pain. Neurologic: No headaches, loss of consciousness, seizures, focal symptoms. Musculoskeletal: No joint swelling, neck pain, back pain. Eyes: No visual changes, painful discharge. ENT: No sore throat, earache, hearing changes. Hematologic: No anemia, abnormal bleeding, nodes, transfusion. Dermatologic: No rash, pruritus, lacerations, contusions. Psychiatric: No depression, A/V hallucinations, suicidal or homicidal ideations. GU: No dysuria, urgency, frequency, hesitancy, nocturia or hematuria. Endocrine: No heat or cold intolerance, no thyroid trouble.

(continued)

s/b *described* for uniformity in tense

s/b *from*, typographical error

s/b *is*, incorrect tense; verb refers to *set* (singular), not to *enzymes* (plural)

s/b *T-wave*, insert hyphen, AAMT Book of Style, hyphens

PAST MEDICAL HISTORY: Positive as noted in HPI.

PAST SURGICAL HISTORY: Negative exact as noted above.

SOCIAL HISTORY: Negative for cigarette or alcohol use.

FAMILY HISTORY: Positive for hypertension.

s/b except, typographical error

MEDICATIONS: Current medications include thalidomide, lactulose, Restoril; Pepcid 20 mg p.o. b.i.d.; Lopressor 12.5 p.o. b.i.d.; Zocor 40 mg p.o. q.h.s.; Medrol 4 mg p.o. q.d.; Norvasc 10 mg a day. The patient is also on Flomax 0.4 mg p.o. q. day; Synthroid 0.025 mg; Imdur 30 mg p.o. q. day; Sinemet 25/100; Senokot; Coumadin 3 mg a day; Lasix 20 mg p.o. q. day.

s/b q. day, ISMP List of Dangerous Abbreviations

PHYSICAL EXAMINATION: A well-developed, well-nourished male, alert and comfortable. Vital signs show a blood pressure of 108/88, pulse of 64 and respiratory rate 18, temperature 98.9. Head was normal shape, no trauma. Eyes: Pupils equal, reactive to light and accommodation. Extraocular motions were intact. ENT: Nondeformed nose, normal lips, teeth and gums. Tongue and palate were clear. External canals were seen. Oral mucosa was moist with no exudate. Neck was supple, nontender, no masses, no JVD, trachea was midline. Cardiovascular: Regular rate and rhythm, with no murmurs, rubs or gallops. No pedal edema. Pulses were equal throughout. Respiratory effort: Lungs were clear to auscultation with no use of accessory muscles, no retractions. Chest: There is some reproducibility of the chest pain. GI: Normal bowel sounds, no masses. GU: Deferred. Musculoskeletal: Three limbs were present, with full range of motion. Back: No spasms, no spinous tenderness. Neurologic: Cranial nerves II through XII were intact. Patient was alert, oriented x3, with normal mental status. No lymphadenopathy appreciated.

LABORATORY DATA: First troponin was 0.03; ECG was described above; creatinine 1.3. White count 4600.

IMPRESSION:
1. History of chest pain.
2. Shortness of breath.
3. Coronary artery disease with multiple stents, reports unavailable.
4. Hypertension.
5. Hyperlipidemia.
6. Multiple myeloma.
7. History of renal artery stent.
8. History of DVT.
9. History of chronic anticoagulation with Coumadin therapy.

s/b deep venous thrombosis or deep vein thrombosis, expand abbreviations in the Impression section of the report, AAMT Book of Style, abbreviations, acronyms, brief forms

(continued)

10. Chronic renal insufficiency.

11. Dementia.

12. History of below-knee amputation.

13. Hypothyroidism.

14. Benign prostatic hypertrophy.

PLAN:
After a long discussion with the patient and his son, we will rule out the patient by serial enzymes and follow. In terms of the subtherapeutic INR, the patient would probably need adjustment in the Coumadin dose.

move to same line as heading for format continuity

For Signature

Report #13

CONSULTATION FOR CHEST PAIN

CONSULTATION

ATTENDING: XXXX

CONSULTANT: XXXX

CHIEF COMPLAINT: Chest pain.

FINDINGS AND RECOMMENDATIONS OF CONSULTANT: The patient is a pleasant 84-year-old gentleman with multiple medical problems. He has a history of multivessel stenting, history of EF of 45% to 50%, with a recent admission for CHF, with elevated BNP, and also a urinary tract infection. According to his son, he was being transported in a van to a nursing home after a visit outside the nursing home and, in the process of transport, the patient developed chest pain. It may be musculoskeletal in nature, but the patient described some heaviness associated with palpitations. He does have a history of coronary disease and has numerous other medical problems as well. He is a fairly poor historian, and most of the information obtained is from the patient's son. In terms of the ECG, he has evidence of T-wave inversions seen in I and aVL. His first set of enzymes is pending. The patient also has severe peripheral vascular disease, has a history of chronic constipation, has a history of renal insufficiency, multiple myeloma as well and has had a history of a left lower extremity DVT leading to being placed on chronic anticoagulation. He also has a history of anemia and has had prior GI workup, the records of which are unavailable at this time. Patient describes some reproducible chest pain with palpation, but no diaphoresis and no radiation of the pain to the back; no orthopnea or PND.

REVIEW OF SYSTEMS: General: No fevers, chills, weight loss or weakness. Cardiovascular: See the HPI. Respiratory: See the HPI. GI: No nausea, vomiting, diarrhea; no abdominal pain or GI pain. Neurologic: No headaches, loss of consciousness, seizures, focal symptoms. Musculoskeletal: No joint swelling, neck pain, back pain. Eyes: No visual changes, painful discharge. ENT: No sore throat, earache, hearing changes. Hematologic: No anemia, abnormal bleeding, nodes, transfusion. Dermatologic: No rash, pruritus, lacerations, contusions. Psychiatric: No depression, A/V hallucinations, suicidal or homicidal ideations. GU: No dysuria, urgency, frequency, hesitancy, nocturia or hematuria. Endocrine: No heat or cold intolerance, no thyroid trouble.

PAST MEDICAL HISTORY: Positive as noted in HPI.

PAST SURGICAL HISTORY: Negative except as noted above.

SOCIAL HISTORY: Negative for cigarette or alcohol use.

FAMILY HISTORY: Positive for hypertension.

(continued)

MEDICATIONS: Current medications include thalidomide, lactulose, Restoril; Pepcid 20 mg p.o. b.i.d.; Lopressor 12.5 p.o. b.i.d.; Zocor 40 mg p.o. q.h.s.; Medrol 4 mg p.o. q. day; Norvasc 10 mg a day. The patient is also on Flomax 0.4 mg p.o. q. day; Synthroid 0.025 mg; Imdur 30 mg p.o. q. day; Sinemet 25/100; Senokot; Coumadin 3 mg a day; Lasix 20 mg p.o. q. day.

PHYSICAL EXAMINATION: A well-developed, well-nourished male, alert and comfortable. Vital signs show a blood pressure of 108/88, pulse of 64 and respiratory rate 18, temperature 98.9. Head was normal shape, no trauma. Eyes: Pupils equal, reactive to light and accommodation. Extraocular motions were intact. ENT: Nondeformed nose, normal lips, teeth and gums. Tongue and palate were clear. External canals were seen. Oral mucosa was moist with no exudate. Neck was supple, nontender, no masses, no JVD, trachea was midline. Cardiovascular: Regular rate and rhythm, with no murmurs, rubs or gallops. No pedal edema. Pulses were equal throughout. Respiratory effort: Lungs were clear to auscultation with no use of accessory muscles, no retractions. Chest: There is some reproducibility of the chest pain. GI: Normal bowel sounds, no masses. GU: Deferred. Musculoskeletal: Three limbs were present, with full range of motion. Back: No spasms, no spinous tenderness. Neurologic: Cranial nerves II through XII were intact. Patient was alert, oriented x3, with normal mental status. No lymphadenopathy appreciated.

LABORATORY DATA: First troponin was 0.03; ECG was described above; creatinine 1.3. White count 4600.

IMPRESSION:
1. History of chest pain.
2. Shortness of breath.
3. Coronary artery disease with multiple stents, reports unavailable.
4. Hypertension.
5. Hyperlipidemia.
6. Multiple myeloma.
7. History of renal artery stent.
8. History of deep venous thrombosis.
9. History of chronic anticoagulation with Coumadin therapy.
10. Chronic renal insufficiency.
11. Dementia.
12. History of below-knee amputation.
13. Hypothyroidism.
14. Benign prostatic hypertrophy.

PLAN: After a long discussion with the patient and his son, we will rule out the patient by serial enzymes and follow. In terms of the subtherapeutic INR, the patient would probably need adjustment in the Coumadin dose.

Answer Key

Report #14

NORMAL THALLIUM STRESS TEST

CARDIAC IMAGING

PROCEDURE

Thallium stress test.

INDICATIONS

This is a 51-year-old with chest pain.

Baseline ECG shows normal sinus rhythm.

s/b showed for uniformity in tense

Patient underwent a treadmill stress test according to the standard Bruce protocol, exercising for 9 minutes, achieving a maximum heart rate of 143 beats per minute, which is greater than 85% of the target heart rate.

SYMPTOMS

No chest pain reported, no ECG changes noted.

Maximum blood pressure attained 200/100, a slightly hypertensive response, which is probably related to deconditioning.

No arrhythmias were noted. The recovery phase was uneventful. Approximately one minute prior to termination of the study, and at peak exercise, the patient was injected with thallium chloride intravenously, subsequently underwent nuclear imaging.

CONCLUSION

1. No electrocardiographic changes noted.
2. Low probability.
3. Duke score of 9.
4. No chest pain reported.
5. No arrhythmias noted.
6. Thallium pending at the time of this dictation.

delete comma, insert period and begin new sentence: ...intravenously. Patient subsequently...

For Signature

NORMAL THALLIUM STRESS TEST

CARDIAC IMAGING

PROCEDURE

Thallium stress test.

INDICATIONS

This is a 51-year-old with chest pain.

Baseline ECG showed normal sinus rhythm.

Patient underwent a treadmill stress test according to the standard Bruce protocol, exercising for 9 minutes, achieving a maximum heart rate of 143 beats per minute, which is greater than 85% of the target heart rate.

SYMPTOMS

No chest pain reported, no ECG changes noted.

Maximum blood pressure attained 200/100, a slightly hypertensive response, which is probably related to deconditioning.

No arrhythmias were noted. The recovery phase was uneventful. Approximately one minute prior to termination of the study, and at peak exercise, the patient was injected with thallium chloride intravenously. Patient subsequently underwent nuclear imaging.

CONCLUSION

1. No electrocardiographic changes noted.
2. Low probability.
3. Duke score of 9.
4. No chest pain reported.
5. No arrhythmias noted.
6. Thallium pending at the time of this dictation.

Answer Key

CARDIOTHORACIC SURGICAL CONSULTATION FOR EVALUATION OF SUITABILITY FOR BYPASS GRAFT SURGERY

CONSULTATION REPORT

ATTENDING: XXXX

CONSULTANT: XXXX

REASON FOR CONSULTATION: A 62-year-old male with known coronary artery disease, with increasing angina pectoris, for myocardial revascularization.

HISTORY: A 62-year-old male with known coronary artery disease presented with progressive angina pectoris. He has a history of an acute myocardial infarction in October 2003, and has undergone placement of PTCA and stents to the right and diagonal coronary arteries. He also has a history of ventricular tachycardia and has undergone AICD placement. He has been followed by nuclear stress tests and diagnostic catheterizations. He notes increasing frequency of substernal chest pain. His last episode was in September; while exercising, he developed substernal discomfort radiating to his left hand, associated with diaphoresis. His symptoms resolved with two nitroglycerin tablets. Nuclear stress test in October 10, 2005, was noted to be abnormal, by history. Results, unfortunately, are not in the chart. Diagnostic catheterization was performed today, revealing significant 3-vessel coronary artery disease and moderately severe left ventricular dysfunction, with overall ejection fraction in the 30% range. Because of this, we were asked to see him in consultation for surgical opinion.

PAST MEDICAL HISTORY: Pertinent for diabetes, Niaspan intolerance, history of cataracts, hypothyroidism, hypertension.

MEDICATIONS: NovoLog 70/30, 12 units q.a.m., 8 units q.p.m.; hydrochlorothiazide 25 mg. q. day; Synthroid 0.05 mg. q. Tuesday-Thursday-Saturday-Sunday, 0.075 mg. Monday-Wednesday-Friday; amiodarone 100 mg. h.s.; aspirin 81 mg. q. day; Coreg 12.5 mg. b.i.d.; Plavix 75 mg. q. day, which last dose was last night; digoxin 0.25 mg. h.s.; Vasotec 5 mg. b.i.d.; Inspra 25 mg. h.s.; Zocor 40 mg. h.s.; glipizide ER 10 mg. b.i.d.

ALLERGIES: Ibuprofen and Niaspan.

(continued)

Annotations:

alt.: change *A* to *This* for clarity

s/b *on*, typographical error

delete the period after *mg* throughout paragraph, AAMT Book of Style, mg

FAMILY HISTORY: Denies coronary artery disease.

SOCIAL HISTORY: Previous tobacco abuse.

REVIEW OF SYSTEMS: No weight loss, weight gain, fever, chills. No eye pain, double vision; he has a history of cataracts. No eye discharge. No tinnitus, vertigo, frequent sore throats. He reports chest pain, no palpitations, no AICD discharge recently. No lower extremity edema. No hemoptysis, wheezing, pneumonia, or GI bleeding, hepatitis, gallbladder disease. No polyuria, polydipsia, polyphagia. He is on Synthroid. He reports prolonged bleeding secondary to aspirin and Plavix; prior to medications, he had no bleeding disorders. No cellulitis, no skin cancers. No lymphadenopathy. No TIA, amaurosis, frequent headaches. No mood swings, suicide intent, depression. No joint pain, back pain, muscle pain.

alt.: delete or *for uniformity*

substitute face *for clarity*

PHYSICAL EXAMINATION: In general, he is an alert male, on bed rest, in no acute distress. Blood pressure on admission was 120/76, pulse 74, regular; respirations 18 and unlabored; no fever. HEENT: Normocephalic, atraumatic. No deformities to the facial or head. Mucous membranes are moist. No scleral jaundice. Neck supple, with no carotid bruits, no JVD, no thyroid enlargement, nodules or tenderness. No carotid bruits. Lungs had good excursion, no use of accessory muscles; clear to auscultation. Heart: PMI displaced laterally. No palpable thrill. Regular rate and rhythm without murmur. Abdomen soft, nontender. No epigastric bruit, no hepatosplenomegaly, no abdominal aortic aneurysm, no tenderness; bowel sounds present. Extremity examination notes some right femoral artery pressure dressing, left femoral is 4+ without bruit. Popliteals are 3+, pedals are 3+. No clubbing, cyanosis or edema. Good saphenous veins. Musculoskeletal: No scoliosis, joint effusions, muscle wasting. Lymphatics: No supraclavicular, axillary or femoral lymphadenopathy. Neurological examination grossly intact. Motor, sensory and cranial nerves are intact. Oriented x3, to time, personal and place. Affect normal. Skin: No obvious skin lesions, skin cancer, cellulitis. Breasts: No abnormal breast masses. GU: Normal male. No CVA tenderness.

delete entire sentence, repetitive

delete some

LABORATORY DATA: Diagnostic catheterization as noted. WBC 8100, hematocrit 45%, platelet count 180,000. Potassium 4.4, creatinine 1, glucose 231, INR 1.1.

IMPRESSION:

1. Coronary artery disease with:
   • Angina pectoris.
   • History of inferior wall myocardial infarction.

(continued)

- Left ventricular dysfunction.
- Positive nuclear stress test.

2. Diabetes.
3. Previous tobacco abuse.
4. Hypertension.
5. Plavix and aspirin use.
6. Nonsustained ventricular tachycardia, status post automatic implantable cardioverter defibrillator.

PLAN:

Coagulation panel to assess bleeding tendencies. Myocardial revascularization following results of that. Risks, benefits, options, indications and alternatives to surgery have been discussed in detail with patient, family and wife. Following careful discussion and understanding, he has elected to proceed with the operation.

move to same line as heading for format continuity

For Signature

CARDIOTHORACIC SURGICAL CONSULTATION FOR EVALUATION OF SUITABILITY FOR BYPASS GRAFT SURGERY

CONSULTATION REPORT

ATTENDING: XXXX

CONSULTANT: XXXX

REASON FOR CONSULTATION: A 62-year-old male with known coronary artery disease, with increasing angina pectoris, for myocardial revascularization.

HISTORY: This 62-year-old male with known coronary artery disease presented with progressive angina pectoris. He has a history of an acute myocardial infarction in October 2003, and has undergone placement of PTCA and stents to the right and diagonal coronary arteries. He also has a history of ventricular tachycardia and has undergone AICD placement. He has been followed by nuclear stress tests and diagnostic catheterizations. He notes increasing frequency of substernal chest pain. His last episode was in September; while exercising, he developed substernal discomfort radiating to his left hand, associated with diaphoresis. His symptoms resolved with two nitroglycerin tablets. Nuclear stress test on October 10, 2005, was noted to be abnormal, by history. Results, unfortunately, are not in the chart. Diagnostic catheterization was performed today, revealing significant 3-vessel coronary artery disease and moderately severe left ventricular dysfunction, with overall ejection fraction in the 30% range. Because of this, we were asked to see him in consultation for surgical opinion.

PAST MEDICAL HISTORY: Pertinent for diabetes, Niaspan intolerance, history of cataracts, hypothyroidism, hypertension.

MEDICATIONS: NovoLog 70/30, 12 units q.a.m., 8 units q.p.m.; hydrochlorothiazide 25 mg q. day; Synthroid 0.05 mg q. Tuesday-Thursday-Saturday-Sunday, 0.075 mg Monday-Wednesday-Friday; amiodarone 100 mg h.s.; aspirin 81 mg q. day; Coreg 12.5 mg b.i.d.; Plavix 75 mg q. day, which last dose was last night; digoxin 0.25 mg h.s.; Vasotec 5 mg b.i.d.; Inspra 25 mg h.s.; Zocor 40 mg h.s.; glipizide ER 10 mg b.i.d.

ALLERGIES: Ibuprofen and Niaspan.

FAMILY HISTORY: Denies coronary artery disease.

SOCIAL HISTORY: Previous tobacco abuse.

REVIEW OF SYSTEMS: No weight loss, weight gain, fever, chills. No eye pain, double vision; he has a history of cataracts. No eye discharge. No tinnitus, vertigo, frequent sore throats. He reports chest pain, no palpitations, no AICD discharge recently. No lower extremity edema. No hemoptysis, wheezing, pneumonia, GI bleeding, hepatitis, gallbladder disease. No polyuria, polydipsia, polyphagia. He is on Synthroid. He reports prolonged bleeding secondary to aspirin

(continued)

and Plavix; prior to medications, he had no bleeding disorders. No cellulitis, no skin cancers. No lymphadenopathy. No TIA, amaurosis, frequent headaches. No mood swings, suicide intent, depression. No joint pain, back pain, muscle pain.

PHYSICAL EXAMINATION: In general, he is an alert male, on bed rest, in no acute distress. Blood pressure on admission was 120/76, pulse 74, regular; respirations 18 and unlabored; no fever. HEENT: Normocephalic, atraumatic. No deformities to the face or head. Mucous membranes are moist. No scleral jaundice. Neck supple, with no carotid bruits, no JVD, no thyroid enlargement, nodules or tenderness. Lungs had good excursion, no use of accessory muscles; clear to auscultation. Heart: PMI displaced laterally. No palpable thrill. Regular rate and rhythm without murmur. Abdomen soft, nontender. No epigastric bruit, no hepatosplenomegaly, no abdominal aortic aneurysm, no tenderness; bowel sounds present. Extremity examination notes right femoral artery pressure dressing, left femoral is 4+ without bruit. Popliteals are 3+, pedals are 3+. No clubbing, cyanosis or edema. Good saphenous veins. Musculoskeletal: No scoliosis, joint effusions, muscle wasting. Lymphatics: No supraclavicular, axillary or femoral lymphadenopathy. Neurological examination grossly intact. Motor, sensory and cranial nerves are intact. Oriented x3, to time, personal and place. Affect normal. Skin: No obvious skin lesions, skin cancer, cellulitis. Breasts: No abnormal breast masses. GU: Normal male. No CVA tenderness.

LABORATORY DATA: Diagnostic catheterization as noted. WBC 8100, hematocrit 45%, platelet count 180,000. Potassium 4.4, creatinine 1, glucose 231, INR 1.1.

IMPRESSION:

1. Coronary artery disease with:
   • Angina pectoris.
   • History of inferior wall myocardial infarction.
   • Left ventricular dysfunction.
   • Positive nuclear stress test.
2. Diabetes.
3. Previous tobacco abuse.
4. Hypertension.
5. Plavix and aspirin use.
6. Nonsustained ventricular tachycardia, status post automatic implantable cardioverter defibrillator.

PLAN: Coagulation panel to assess bleeding tendencies. Myocardial revascularization following results of that. Risks, benefits, options, indications and alternatives to surgery have been discussed in detail with patient, family and wife. Following careful discussion and understanding, he has elected to proceed with the operation.

Answer Key

CONSULTATION FOR PATIENT WITH PERICARDITIS

CONSULTATION

ATTENDING:

XXXX

CONSULTANT:

XXXX

FINDINGS AND RECOMMENDATIONS OF CONSULTANT:

IMPRESSION:

1. Pericarditis with electrocardiographic changes consistent with pericarditis and pleuritic chest pain; respiratory tract infection approximately a month ago.
2. Occasional tobacco use.
3. Positive family history for coronary artery disease.

PLAN/RECOMMENDATION:

Obtain serial cardiac enzymes and EEGs; 2-D echocardiography to evaluate left ventricular systolic function. If enzymes are negative, then proceed with treadmill stress testing.

The patient is a 33-year-old male who was in his usual state of health up until a week ago when he began developing chest discomfort with inspiration. However, on the morning of admission, he woke up with stabbing chest pain, worsened by inspiration, but not with moving or palpation. With the pain persisting, patient sought medical attention at the emergency room where he was evaluated and subsequently admitted. His pain went away with analgesics. Patient denies a history of coronary artery disease in the past, has never had cardiac testing. No congestive heart failure, valvular or rheumatic heart disease.

CARDIAC RISK FACTORS:

Occasional tobacco use, but no dyslipidemia, diabetes or hypertension.

FAMILY HISTORY:

Questionable. He states his father died of a myocardial infarction at the age of 30?

(continued)

s/b *ECGs* or *EKGs*, typographical error

insert heading of *HISTORY:* or *HISTORY OF PRESENT ILLNESS:* for report uniformity

REVIEW OF SYSTEMS:

Significant for above. History of genital herpes. Denies CVA, seizure disorder, thyroid disease, asthma, bronchitis, emphysema, peptic ulcer disease or GI bleeding, viral hepatitis or pancreatitis, change in bowel habits, involuntary weight loss, kidney stones, renal insufficiency, gout, DVT, claudication, pulmonary embolism or malignancies.

PAST SURGICAL HISTORY:

Status post appendectomy in childhood.

ALLERGIES:

No known drug allergies.

MEDICATIONS:

Prior to admission, Valtrex.

SOCIAL HISTORY:

No alcohol or drug abuse. He is a smoker, smoking a few cigarettes occasionally.

PHYSICAL EXAMINATION:

Physical examination reveals a well-developed, well-nourished male, in no apparent distress. Vital signs: Blood pressure is 130/70, pulse is 18 and regular, respiratory rate 80. HEENT atraumatic, normocephalic. Anicteric sclerae. Neck veins not distended at a 30-degree angle, carotid upstrokes not delayed, no bruits. Lungs are clear to auscultation and percussion. PMI is not displaced, first and second heart sounds are regular without gallops or murmurs. Abdomen is soft, nontender, with normoactive bowel sounds. No visceromegaly, masses or bruits. Extremities without edema, cyanosis or clubbing. Peripheral pulses are intact.

s/b pulse 80, respiratory rate 18, NOTE: pulse and respiration values are commonly transposed in dictation

LABORATORY DATA:

Sodium 141, potassium 3.7, BUN 18, creatinine 0.9. Cardiac enzymes x2 negative for myocardial necrosis. WBC on admission was 12,100, but this morning 6,800; hemoglobin 14.7, hematocrit 42.3%, platelet count 279,000. D-dimer was normal at 0.7. Chest x-ray reported as normal, will review.

For Signature

CONSULTATION FOR PATIENT WITH PERICARDITIS

CONSULTATION

ATTENDING:

 XXXX

CONSULTANT:

XXXX

FINDINGS AND RECOMMENDATIONS OF CONSULTANT:

IMPRESSION:

1. Pericarditis with electrocardiographic changes consistent with pericarditis and pleuritic chest pain; respiratory tract infection approximately a month ago.
2. Occasional tobacco use.
3. Positive family history for coronary artery disease.

PLAN/RECOMMENDATION:

Obtain serial cardiac enzymes and EKGs; 2-D echocardiography to evaluate left ventricular systolic function. If enzymes are negative, then proceed with treadmill stress testing.

HISTORY:

The patient is a 33-year-old male who was in his usual state of health up until a week ago when he began developing chest discomfort with inspiration. However, on the morning of admission, he woke up with stabbing chest pain, worsened by inspiration, but not with moving or palpation. With the pain persisting, patient sought medical attention at the emergency room where he was evaluated and subsequently admitted. His pain went away with analgesics. Patient denies a history of coronary artery disease in the past, has never had cardiac testing. No congestive heart failure, valvular or rheumatic heart disease.

CARDIAC RISK FACTORS:

Occasional tobacco use, but no dyslipidemia, diabetes or hypertension.

FAMILY HISTORY:

Questionable. He states his father died of a myocardial infarction at the age of 30?

REVIEW OF SYSTEMS:

Significant for above. History of genital herpes. Denies CVA, seizure disorder, thyroid disease, asthma, bronchitis, emphysema, peptic ulcer disease or GI bleeding, viral hepatitis or pancreatitis, change in bowel habits, involuntary weight loss, kidney stones, renal insufficiency, gout, DVT, claudication, pulmonary embolism or malignancies.

(continued)

PAST SURGICAL HISTORY:

Status post appendectomy in childhood.

ALLERGIES:

No known drug allergies.

MEDICATIONS:

Prior to admission, Valtrex.

SOCIAL HISTORY:

No alcohol or drug abuse. He is a smoker, smoking a few cigarettes occasionally.

PHYSICAL EXAMINATION:

Physical examination reveals a well-developed, well-nourished male, in no apparent distress. Vital signs: Blood pressure is 130/70, pulse is 80 and regular, respiratory rate 18. HEENT atraumatic, normocephalic. Anicteric sclerae. Neck veins not distended at a 30-degree angle, carotid upstrokes not delayed, no bruits. Lungs are clear to auscultation and percussion. PMI is not displaced, first and second heart sounds are regular without gallops or murmurs. Abdomen is soft, nontender, with normoactive bowel sounds. No visceromegaly, masses or bruits. Extremities without edema, cyanosis or clubbing. Peripheral pulses are intact.

LABORATORY DATA:

Sodium 141, potassium 3.7, BUN 18, creatinine 0.9. Cardiac enzymes x2 negative for myocardial necrosis. WBC on admission was 12,100, but this morning 6,800; hemoglobin 14.7, hematocrit 42.3%, platelet count 279,000. D-dimer was normal at 0.7. Chest x-ray reported as normal, will review.

Answer Key

ABNORMAL TRANSESOPHAGEAL ECHOCARDIOGRAM

ECHOCARDIOGRAM STUDY

PROCEDURE: Transesophageal echocardiogram.

INDICATIONS: A 73-year-old female with rheumatic heart disease, history of mitral valve prolapse, and recently documented echocardiogram suggesting possible ruptured chordae with moderate to severe mitral regurgitation reported.

LOCAL ANESTHETIC: Cetacaine spray 10%.

INTRAVENOUS SEDATION: Versed 4 mg and Demerol 50 mcg.

s/b mg, dosage incorrect, Quick Look Drug Book 2006, meperidine

PROCEDURE DETAILS: Consent was obtained for a transesophageal echocardiogram study. The risks and the benefits of the procedure were explained to the patient in detail. The patient was placed in the left lateral decubitus position and after appropriate sedation and local anesthetic were given. While under constant heart rate, blood pressure and pulse oximetry monitoring, the OmniPlane transesophageal echocardiogram probe was inserted via the posterior pharynx into the esophagus, with multiple views obtained. Subsequently, the probe was removed without difficulty. The patient tolerated the procedure well, with no apparent complications.

delete and

FINDINGS: The left ventricle is normal in size, internal dimensions and wall thickness. The ventricle is only partially visualized in the TEE view, due to the heart beating off axis. Right ventricle is normal in size and function. The left and right atrium are mildly dilated. The interatrial septum is intact. Color flow study across the interatrial septum demonstrates no evidence of right-to-left or left-to-right shunting. Left atrial appendage is partially visualized and appears to be unremarkable. Mitral valve is structurally abnormal. The mitral valve anterior leaflet is thickened and myxomatous; it demonstrates prolapse. There are two separate jets of mitral regurgitation noted, demonstrating moderate mitral regurgitation. No stenosis is seen. There is no evidence for ruptured chordae. The aortic valve leaflets are visualized. They are grossly trileaflet; they are mildly thickened. The aortic valve leaflets open without stenosis and close without prolapse. Pulmonic and tricuspid valves appear unremarkable. There is evidence for mild tricuspid regurgitation. No pericardial effusion is seen. There is mild to moderate atherosclerotic plaquing of the

s/b atria, stating both left and right makes this plural

(continued)

thoracic aorta. The ascending and descending aorta appears essentially normal.

CONCLUSION:
1. Normal left ventricular size and systolic function.
2. Mitral valve prolapse with moderate mitral regurgitation. No evidence for ruptured chordae.
3. Mildly thickened aortic valve leaflets with associated mild aortic regurgitation.
4. Remaining valves are structurally unremarkable.
5. No thrombus or vegetation is identified.
6. No pericardial effusion is seen.
7. Mild to moderate atherosclerotic plaquing of the thoracic descending aorta is seen.

For Signature

ABNORMAL TRANSESOPHAGEAL ECHOCARDIOGRAM

ECHOCARDIOGRAM STUDY

PROCEDURE: Transesophageal echocardiogram.

INDICATIONS: A 73-year-old female with rheumatic heart disease, history of mitral valve prolapse, and recently documented echocardiogram suggesting possible ruptured chordae with moderate to severe mitral regurgitation reported.

LOCAL ANESTHETIC: Cetacaine spray 10%.

INTRAVENOUS SEDATION: Versed 4 mg and Demerol 50 mg.

PROCEDURE DETAILS: Consent was obtained for a transesophageal echocardiogram study. The risks and the benefits of the procedure were explained to the patient in detail. The patient was placed in the left lateral decubitus position after appropriate sedation and local anesthetic were given. While under constant heart rate, blood pressure and pulse oximetry monitoring, the OmniPlane transesophageal echocardiogram probe was inserted via the posterior pharynx into the esophagus, with multiple views obtained. Subsequently, the probe was removed without difficulty. The patient tolerated the procedure well, with no apparent complications.

FINDINGS: The left ventricle is normal in size, internal dimensions and wall thickness. The ventricle is only partially visualized in the TEE view, due to the heart beating off axis. Right ventricle is normal in size and function. The left and right atria are mildly dilated. The interatrial septum is intact. Color flow study across the interatrial septum demonstrates no evidence of right-to-left or left-to-right shunting. Left atrial appendage is partially visualized and appears to be unremarkable. Mitral valve is structurally abnormal. The mitral valve anterior leaflet is thickened and myxomatous; it demonstrates prolapse. There are two separate jets of mitral regurgitation noted, demonstrating moderate mitral regurgitation. No stenosis is seen. There is no evidence for ruptured chordae. The aortic valve leaflets are visualized. They are grossly trileaflet; they are mildly thickened. The aortic valve leaflets open without stenosis and close without prolapse. Pulmonic and tricuspid valves appear unremarkable. There is evidence for mild tricuspid regurgitation. No pericardial effusion is seen. There is mild to moderate atherosclerotic plaquing of the thoracic aorta. The ascending and descending aorta appears essentially normal.

CONCLUSION:
1. Normal left ventricular size and systolic function.
2. Mitral valve prolapse with moderate mitral regurgitation. No evidence for ruptured chordae.
3. Mildly thickened aortic valve leaflets with associated mild aortic regurgitation.
4. Remaining valves are structurally unremarkable.
5. No thrombus or vegetation is identified.
6. No pericardial effusion is seen.
7. Mild to moderate atherosclerotic plaquing of the thoracic descending aorta is seen.

Answer Key

Report #18

CONSULTATION FOR PATIENT WITH HEART MURMUR (PEDIATRIC)

CONSULTATION REPORT

REQUESTING: XXXX

CONSULTANT: XXXX

REASON FOR CONSULTATION: I was asked to evaluate this baby boy because of the finding of heart murmur.

This is a 2-day-old male newborn who was born by cesarean section delivery because of previous C-section. His Apgar scores were 8 at one minute and 9 at five minutes. He required oxygenation right after delivery because of mild respiratory distress that was thought to be transient tachypnea of the neonate. His birth weight was 3.178 kg. He is now asymptomatic from a cardiovascular standpoint. There is no history of pallor, cyanosis, easy fatigability or syncope. He is progressing nicely with p.o. enteral feedings. He is on ampicillin and gentamicin because of his respiratory distress soon after delivery. His blood cultures are negative at 48 hours. His CBC is normal. His chest x-ray is normal as well. Heart murmur was heard today on physical examination and thought to be compatible with a holosystolic murmur, likely a ventricular septal defect. Cardiac consultation was requested.

s/b flagged for physician to review for accuracy of statement; appears to be dictated more by rote than as a logical finding in a 2-day-old

He is the third child of a 25-year-old mom. His older siblings are healthy. His family history is negative for congenital heart disease or sudden death.

s/b mother, AAMT Book of Style, family relationship names

Physical examination revealed a full-term newborn, active and alert, with a weight of 3035 gm. His temperature was 98.5, heart rate was 148 per minute, respiratory rat was 38 per minute and unlabored. His oxygen saturation was 96% on room air. His blood pressure was obtained in all four extremities. The right arm was 64/42, right leg 75/50, left arm 78/44, and left leg 78/42 mmHg. His mucous membranes were moist and pink. Bruits were not auscultated. His carotid pulses were strong and symmetric. JVD was not seen. His thyroid gland was not palpable. Adenopathies were not palpated. His lungs were clear to auscultation. Bilateral breath sounds were heard. His precordium was normally active on chest exam. The first and second heart sounds were both normal; a grade 3/6 holosystolic

s/b rate, typographical error

(continued)

murmur was heard at the left sternal border, radiating over the precordium. Diastolic murmurs were not heard. Clicks were not heard. His abdomen was soft; his liver was 1 cm below the costal margin. Organomegaly was not palpated. Abdominal bruits were not heard. Normal male genitalia was noted. His peripheral pulses were strong and symmetric, without brachial-femoral delay noted. Peripheral edema was not seen.

s/b were, plural

An ECG demonstrated sinus rhythm with normal intervals for age. Right axis deviation with right ventricular prominence was noted; that is a normal finding for a neonate. A cardiac ultrasound was reviewed and interpreted by me. It demonstrated a patent foramen ovale and trivial left peripheral branch pulmonic stenosis, which are physiologic findings for age. Additionally, a small (2- to 3-mm) mid muscular ventricular septal defect with left-to-right shunt was noted. The aortic arch was normal. PDA was not seen.

s/b mid-muscular, modifying adjective, AAMT Book of Style, hyphens

SUMMARY:

move to same line as heading for format continuity

In summary, this newborn's evaluation is consistent with a small ventricular septal defect of no hemodynamic significance at this point. My only recommendation is bacterial endocarditis prophylaxis when at risk for bacteremia, and a follow-up appointment in the outpatient cardiac clinic in approximately 3 months. The findings were communicated to his mother and the attending physician.

Thanks for this consultation.

For Signature

CONSULTATION FOR PATIENT WITH HEART MURMUR (PEDIATRIC)

FLAG: Please clarify accuracy of description used in first page, second paragraph under REASON FOR CONSULTATION, 6th line: "easy fatigability". Thank you.

CONSULTATION REPORT

REQUESTING: XXXX

CONSULTANT: XXXX

REASON FOR CONSULTATION: I was asked to evaluate this baby boy because of the finding of heart murmur.

This is a 2-day-old male newborn who was born by cesarean section delivery because of previous C-section. His Apgar scores were 8 at one minute and 9 at five minutes. He required oxygenation right after delivery because of mild respiratory distress that was thought to be transient tachypnea of the neonate. His birth weight was 3.178 kg. He is now asymptomatic from a cardiovascular standpoint. There is no history of pallor, cyanosis, _easy fatigability_ or syncope. He is progressing nicely with p.o. enteral feedings. He is on ampicillin and gentamicin because of his respiratory distress soon after delivery. His blood cultures are negative at 48 hours. His CBC is normal. His chest x-ray is normal as well. Heart murmur was heard today on physical examination and thought to be compatible with a holosystolic murmur, likely a ventricular septal defect. Cardiac consultation was requested.

He is the third child of a 25-year-old mother. His older siblings are healthy. His family history is negative for congenital heart disease or sudden death.

Physical examination revealed a full-term newborn, active and alert, with a weight of 3035 gm. His temperature was 98.5, heart rate was 148 per minute, respiratory rate was 38 per minute and unlabored. His oxygen saturation was 96% on room air. His blood pressure was obtained in all four extremities. The right arm was 64/42, right leg 75/50, left arm 78/44, and left leg 78/42 mmHg. His mucous membranes were moist and pink. Bruits were not auscultated. His carotid pulses were strong and symmetric. JVD was not seen. His thyroid gland was not palpable. Adenopathies were not palpated. His lungs were clear to auscultation. Bilateral breath sounds were heard. His precordium was normally active on chest exam. The first and second heart sounds were both normal; a grade 3/6 holosystolic murmur was heard at the left sternal border, radiating over the precordium. Diastolic murmurs were not heard. Clicks were not heard. His abdomen was soft; his liver was 1 cm below the costal margin. Organomegaly was not palpated. Abdominal bruits were not heard. Normal male genitalia were noted. His peripheral pulses were strong and symmetric, without brachial-femoral delay noted. Peripheral edema was not seen.

An ECG demonstrated sinus rhythm with normal intervals for age. Right axis deviation with right ventricular prominence was noted; that is a normal finding for a neonate. A cardiac ultrasound was reviewed and interpreted by me. It demonstrated a patent foramen ovale and trivial left

(continued)

peripheral branch pulmonic stenosis, which are physiologic findings for age. Additionally, a small (2- to 3-mm) mid-muscular ventricular septal defect with left-to-right shunt was noted. The aortic arch was normal. PDA was not seen.

SUMMARY: In summary, this newborn's evaluation is consistent with a small ventricular septal defect of no hemodynamic significance at this point. My only recommendation is bacterial endocarditis prophylaxis when at risk for bacteremia, and a follow-up appointment in the outpatient cardiac clinic in approximately 3 months. The findings were communicated to his mother and the attending physician.

Thanks for this consultation.

Answer Key

TILT TABLE TEST

TILT TABLE STUDY

PROCEDURE
Tilt table study.

CLINICAL HISTORY
A very pleasant 88-year-old woman with recurrent syncope and recent myocardial infarction.

DESCRIPTION
The patient underwent tilt table testing on a tilt table with a foot board for weight bearing. Baseline heart rate and blood pressure determinations were made. After being in the upright position for roughly 10 minutes without symptoms or hemodynamic abnormalities, one spray of sublingual nitroglycerin was administered. During this time period, she had reproduction of clinical symptoms with near-syncope as well as sudden and profound drop in systolic blood pressure to 50 mmHg. No significant bradycardia was noted. The table was brought back down to horizontal. She tolerated the procedure quite well.

FINDINGS
1. No pathologic pauses with right-sided or left-sided coronary sinus massage.
2. Positive study for neurocardiogenic syncope with primary vasodepressor component with reproduction of symptoms.

s/b carotid, see Stedman's Medical Dictionary, 28E, for definitions of sinus carotid and sinus coronary

RECOMMENDATIONS
Given these findings, I recommend reinstitution of surgical compression stockings. Will add Florinef 0.1 mg daily therapy. Will discuss these with her cardiologist.

For Signature

TILT TABLE TEST

TILT TABLE STUDY

PROCEDURE
Tilt table study.

CLINICAL HISTORY
A very pleasant 88-year-old woman with recurrent syncope and recent myocardial infarction.

DESCRIPTION
The patient underwent tilt table testing on a tilt table with a foot board for weight bearing. Baseline heart rate and blood pressure determinations were made. After being in the upright position for roughly 10 minutes without symptoms or hemodynamic abnormalities, one spray of sublingual nitroglycerin was administered. During this time period, she had reproduction of clinical symptoms with near-syncope as well as sudden and profound drop in systolic blood pressure to 50 mmHg. No significant bradycardia was noted. The table was brought back down to horizontal. She tolerated the procedure quite well.

FINDINGS
1. No pathologic pauses with right-sided or left-sided carotid sinus massage.
2. Positive study for neurocardiogenic syncope with primary vasodepressor component with reproduction of symptoms.

RECOMMENDATIONS
Given these findings, I recommend reinstitution of surgical compression stockings. Will add Florinef 0.1 mg daily therapy. Will discuss these with her cardiologist.

Answer Key

Report #20

STENTING OF LEFT ANTERIOR DESCENDING ARTERY

PERCUTANEOUS CORONARY INTERVENTION

PROCEDURE: Stenting of proximal left anterior descending with 3.5 x 8-mm Cypher drug-eluting stent. Stenting of mid left anterior descending with 3 x 18-mm Cypher drug-eluting stent. Intracoronary nitroglycerin for spasm.

CLINICAL HISTORY: Patient is a 69-year-old female with a history of coronary artery disease, for stenting of LAD.

DESCRIPTION: Consent was obtained after explaining the risks, benefits and alternatives, risks involving renal failure, retroperitoneal hemorrhage, bleeding, stroke and imponderables. A 7-French sheath was placed in the right femoral artery. An XB 3.5 guide was used to cannulate the left main. An IQ wire was placed in the distal LAD. Nitroglycerin 200 mcg was given to diffuse spasm. Angiomax was administered; patient was already on aspirin and Plavix.

s/b defuse, misspelled

This was followed by primary stenting of proximal LAD with a 3.5 x 8-mm Cypher drug-eluting stent which was employed to 14 atmospheres. Stenosis was reduced from 70% to 0%. The mid LAD was stented with a 3 x 18-mm Cypher drug-eluting stent which was employed to 18 atmospheres. Stenosis was reduced from 70% to 0%. No evidence of any dissection or embolization. Excellent results.

s/b deployed, incorrect term

IMPRESSION: Successful stenting of proximal and mid left anterior descending artery with Cypher drug-eluting stents, with excellent results.

For Signature

STENTING OF LEFT ANTERIOR DESCENDING ARTERY

PERCUTANEOUS CORONARY INTERVENTION

PROCEDURE: Stenting of proximal left anterior descending with 3.5 x 8-mm Cypher drug-eluting stent. Stenting of mid left anterior descending with 3 x 18-mm Cypher drug-eluting stent. Intracoronary nitroglycerin for spasm.

CLINICAL HISTORY: Patient is a 69-year-old female with a history of coronary artery disease, for stenting of LAD.

DESCRIPTION: Consent was obtained after explaining the risks, benefits and alternatives, risks involving renal failure, retroperitoneal hemorrhage, bleeding, stroke and imponderables. A 7-French sheath was placed in the right femoral artery. An XB 3.5 guide was used to cannulate the left main. An IQ wire was placed in the distal LAD. Nitroglycerin 200 mcg was given to defuse spasm. Angiomax was administered; patient was already on aspirin and Plavix.

This was followed by primary stenting of proximal LAD with a 3.5 x 8-mm Cypher drug-eluting stent which was deployed to 14 atmospheres. Stenosis was reduced from 70% to 0%. The mid LAD was stented with a 3 x 18-mm Cypher drug-eluting stent which was deployed to 18 atmospheres. Stenosis was reduced from 70% to 0%. No evidence of any dissection or embolization. Excellent results.

IMPRESSION: Successful stenting of proximal and mid left anterior descending artery with Cypher drug-eluting stents, with excellent results.

Answer Key

Report #21

LEFT HEART CATHETERIZATION AND VENTRICULOGRAPHY IN PATIENT WITH CARDIOMYOPATHY

OPERATIVE REPORT

PROCEDURE: Left heart catheterization, ventriculogram.

INDICATIONS: A 65-year-old admitted with chest pain, positive troponins, stress test showing ischemia.

DESCRIPTION: After informed consent was obtained, the patient was brought to the cardiac catheterization laboratory where the right groin was prepped and draped in the usual sterile fashion. Local anesthesia was achieved using 1% lidocaine. Seldinger technique was used to cannulate the right femoral artery. We used a 5-French system, JL4, JR4, angled pigtail for single-plane ventriculogram. The patient tolerated the procedure without complications.

HEMODYNAMIC FINDINGS: The aortic pressure was 135/77. The LV was 135 with an end-diastolic of 14. There was no gradient on pullback across the aortic valve.

ANGIOGRAPHIC FINDINGS:

LEFT MAIN CORONARY ARTERY: The left main was free of significant disease.

CIRCUMFLEX: The circumflex was a moderate-sized vessel giving off two marginal branches. The did not appear to be significant disease involving these vessels.

s/b There, typographical error

LEFT ANTERIOR DESCENDING: The LAD was a moderate-sized vessel giving off three diagonal branches. The first diagonal was moderate in size; second and third were quite small. There did not appear to be any evidence of significant disease involving the LAD or diagonal system.

s/b focal, typographical error

RIGHT CORONARY ARTERY: The right coronary artery was a moderate-sized vessel, giving off a PDA and a PL branch, both with minimal irregularity. The distal PDA and PL branch are small, but no significant vocal stenosis was appreciated.

s/b were for uniformity in tense

s/b single-plane, adjectival phrase modifying ventriculogram, AAMT Book of Style, hyphens

VENTRICULOGRAM: Single plane ventriculogram showed the ejection fraction was significantly impaired at about 35%.

(continued)

CONCLUSION:

1. Minimal coronary artery disease.
2. Elevated left ventricular end-diastolic pressure.
3. Moderate left ventricular dysfunction, ejection fraction 35%.

RECOMMENDATIONS: This patient appears to have a nonischemic cardiomyopathy. The interesting fact is that her daughter also has cardiomyopathy and required defibrillator placement. Hopefully her ventricle will stabilize with ACE-inhibitor and beta-blocker therapy.

For Signature

LEFT HEART CATHETERIZATION AND VENTRICULOGRAPHY IN PATIENT WITH CARDIOMYOPATHY

OPERATIVE REPORT

PROCEDURE: Left heart catheterization, ventriculogram.

INDICATIONS: A 65-year-old admitted with chest pain, positive troponins, stress test showing ischemia.

DESCRIPTION: After informed consent was obtained, the patient was brought to the cardiac catheterization laboratory where the right groin was prepped and draped in the usual sterile fashion. Local anesthesia was achieved using 1% lidocaine. Seldinger technique was used to cannulate the right femoral artery. We used a 5-French system, JL4, JR4, angled pigtail for single-plane ventriculogram. The patient tolerated the procedure without complications.

HEMODYNAMIC FINDINGS: The aortic pressure was 135/77. The LV was 135 with an end-diastolic of 14. There was no gradient on pullback across the aortic valve.

ANGIOGRAPHIC FINDINGS:

LEFT MAIN CORONARY ARTERY: The left main was free of significant disease.

CIRCUMFLEX: The circumflex was a moderate-sized vessel giving off two marginal branches. There did not appear to be significant disease involving these vessels.

LEFT ANTERIOR DESCENDING: The LAD was a moderate-sized vessel giving off three diagonal branches. The first diagonal was moderate in size; second and third were quite small. There did not appear to be any evidence of significant disease involving the LAD or diagonal system.

RIGHT CORONARY ARTERY: The right coronary artery was a moderate-sized vessel, giving off a PDA and a PL branch, both with minimal irregularity. The distal PDA and PL branch were small, but no significant focal stenosis was appreciated.

VENTRICULOGRAM: Single-plane ventriculogram showed the ejection fraction was significantly impaired at about 35%.

CONCLUSION:
1. Minimal coronary artery disease.
2. Elevated left ventricular end-diastolic pressure.
3. Moderate left ventricular dysfunction, ejection fraction 35%.

RECOMMENDATIONS: This patient appears to have a nonischemic cardiomyopathy. The interesting fact is that her daughter also has cardiomyopathy and required defibrillator placement. Hopefully her ventricle will stabilize with ACE-inhibitor and beta-blocker therapy.

Answer Key

DOBUTAMINE STRESS ECHOCARDIOGRAM

CARDIAC IMAGING

PROCEDURE: Dobutamine stress echocardiogram.

INDICATION: The patient is a 34-year-old female with chest pain. The patient was unable to have a nuclear stress test due to a recent menstrual cycle and, therefore, a dobutamine stress echocardiogram was recommended.

PROTOCOL: After informed consent was obtained, the patient was infused with IV dobutamine starting at 5 mcg/kg/min, increased to a total of 30 mcg/kg/min. The patient was given 0.5 mg of IV atropine to achieve the peak heart rate needed. Her peak heart rate was approximately 160 beats per minute. Peak blood pressure was approximately 150/72. She did have some chest pain and shortness of breath during the protocol.

> change /min to *per minute*; avoid using more than one virgule per expression, AAMT Book of Style, virgule (/)

ELECTROCARDIOGRAPHIC EVALUATION: At baseline, the patient had an ECG which revealed a normal sinus rhythm, nonspecific ST-T wave changes in the inferolateral leads. During peak heart rate, the patient had less than 1 mm of horizontal ST-segment depression. There were no malignant atrial or ventricular arrhythmias noted.

ECHOCARDIOGRAPHIC EVALUATION: Two-dimensional and Doppler ultrasonography were performed in the usual manner. At baseline, the patient had grossly normal left ventricular size and wall thickness with left ventricular ejection fraction estimated at approximately 60%. No significant wall motion abnormalities are noted. There was no significant valvular regurgitation noted. The cardiac valves appear to be structurally within normal limits. Optison was used for the apical views. At peak heart rate, the patient had appropriate augmentation of left ventricular systolic function. No significant wall motion abnormalities are noted. There was appropriate decrease in left ventricular size.

> s/b *were* for uniformity in tense

> s/b *appeared* for uniformity in tense

IMPRESSION:
1. No electrocardiographic evidence for ischemia noted.
2. Echocardiographic evaluation reveals no significant wall motion abnormalities. There is an appropriate decrease in left ventricular size.

For Signature

DOBUTAMINE STRESS ECHOCARDIOGRAM

CARDIAC IMAGING

PROCEDURE: Dobutamine stress echocardiogram.

INDICATION: The patient is a 34-year-old female with chest pain. The patient was unable to have a nuclear stress test due to a recent menstrual cycle and, therefore, a dobutamine stress echocardiogram was recommended.

PROTOCOL: After informed consent was obtained, the patient was infused with IV dobutamine starting at 5 mcg/kg per minute, increased to a total of 30 mcg/kg per minute. The patient was given 0.5 mg of IV atropine to achieve the peak heart rate needed. Her peak heart rate was approximately 160 beats per minute. Peak blood pressure was approximately 150/72. She did have some chest pain and shortness of breath during the protocol.

ELECTROCARDIOGRAPHIC EVALUATION: At baseline, the patient had an ECG which revealed a normal sinus rhythm, nonspecific ST-T wave changes in the inferolateral leads. During peak heart rate, the patient had less than 1 mm of horizontal ST-segment depression. There were no malignant atrial or ventricular arrhythmias noted.

ECHOCARDIOGRAPHIC EVALUATION: Two-dimensional and Doppler ultrasonography were performed in the usual manner. At baseline, the patient had grossly normal left ventricular size and wall thickness with left ventricular ejection fraction estimated at approximately 60%. No significant wall motion abnormalities were noted. There was no significant valvular regurgitation noted. The cardiac valves appeared to be structurally within normal limits. Optison was used for the apical views. At peak heart rate, the patient had appropriate augmentation of left ventricular systolic function. No significant wall motion abnormalities were noted. There was appropriate decrease in left ventricular size.

IMPRESSION:
1. No electrocardiographic evidence for ischemia noted.
2. Echocardiographic evaluation reveals no significant wall motion abnormalities. There is an appropriate decrease in left ventricular size.

Answer Key

ECHOCARDIOGRAM WITH DOPPLER

DOPPLER STUDY

PROCEDURE: Echocardiogram with Doppler.

CLINICAL HISTORY: A 75-year-old man with acute anterior wall myocardial infarction. This study is to evaluate LV function, presence of apical clot, and complications of myocardial infarction.

Procedure of two-dimensional echocardiography, M-mode, and complete Doppler was performed. The quality of the study is good.

FINDINGS:

M-MODE: Left ventricular end-diastolic dimension 3.6 cm, end-systolic dimension 2.7 cm. Interventricular septal thickness 1.7 cm, posterior wall 1.5 cm. Ejection fraction estimated at 45% to 50%. Left atrial size 3.8 cm. Aortic root 3.2 cm.

TWO-DIMENSIONAL: There is a moderate size anteroapical wall motion abnormality. This is moderately to severely hypokinetic, clearly not akinetic. There is no paradoxic motion of the septa. Remaining walls appear to move normally with preserved LV systolic function, ejection fraction around 50%. There is mild mitral annular calcification with mild sclerotic changes of the mitral and aortic valves. The aortic valve is clearly tricuspid, without stenosis. No pericardial effusion is seen. There are no other abnormal calcifications.

DOPPLER: Trace mitral regurgitation is seen, as well as mild tricuspid insufficiency. Pulmonary artery pressure is normal at 33 mmHg. The E-to-A ratio is abnormal, suggesting diastolic noncompliance.

IMPRESSION:
1. Mildly-reduced left ventricular systolic function, ejection fraction 50%, with anteroapical wall motion abnormality, consistent with patient's clinical history of anterior wall myocardial infarction.
2. Mild innocent changes of the mitral and aortic valves, with no hemodynamically significant flow abnormalities.
3. Normal pulmonary pressures.
4. The E-to-A ratio is abnormal, suggesting diastolic noncompliance, which is typical for an infarcted ventricle.
5. No apical clot is identified.

s/b *moderate-size,* hyphenate compound modifiers, AAMT Book of Style, compound modifiers

s/b *septum,* singular

s/b *Mildly reduced;* do not hyphenate modifying adverbs ending in *ly,* AAMT Book of Style, compound modifiers, adverb ending in -ly

s/b *senescent,* incorrect term

For Signature

ECHOCARDIOGRAM WITH DOPPLER

DOPPLER STUDY

PROCEDURE: Echocardiogram with Doppler.

CLINICAL HISTORY: A 75-year-old man with acute anterior wall myocardial infarction. This study is to evaluate LV function, presence of apical clot, and complications of myocardial infarction.

Procedure of two-dimensional echocardiography, M-mode, and complete Doppler was performed. The quality of the study is good.

FINDINGS:

M-MODE: Left ventricular end-diastolic dimension 3.6 cm, end-systolic dimension 2.7 cm. Interventricular septal thickness 1.7 cm, posterior wall 1.5 cm. Ejection fraction estimated at 45% to 50%. Left atrial size 3.8 cm. Aortic root 3.2 cm.

TWO-DIMENSIONAL: There is a moderate-size anteroapical wall motion abnormality. This is moderately to severely hypokinetic, clearly not akinetic. There is no paradoxic motion of the septum. Remaining walls appear to move normally with preserved LV systolic function, ejection fraction around 50%. There is mild mitral annular calcification with mild sclerotic changes of the mitral and aortic valves. The aortic valve is clearly tricuspid, without stenosis. No pericardial effusion is seen. There are no other abnormal calcifications.

DOPPLER: Trace mitral regurgitation is seen, as well as mild tricuspid insufficiency. Pulmonary artery pressure is normal at 33 mmHg. The E-to-A ratio is abnormal, suggesting diastolic noncompliance.

IMPRESSION:
1. Mildly reduced left ventricular systolic function, ejection fraction 50%, with anteroapical wall motion abnormality, consistent with patient's clinical history of anterior wall myocardial infarction.
2. Mild senescent changes of the mitral and aortic valves, with no hemodynamically significant flow abnormalities.
3. Normal pulmonary pressures.
4. The E-to-A ratio is abnormal, suggesting diastolic noncompliance, which is typical for an infarcted ventricle.
5. No apical clot is identified.

Answer Key

PACEMAKER INSERTION (PEDIATRIC)

PACEMAKER REPORT

PREOPERATIVE DIAGNOSIS:
1. Status post repair of pulmonary atresia and tetralogy of Fallot.
2. Third-degree heart block.

POSTOPERATIVE DIAGNOSIS:
1. Status post repair of pulmonary atresia and tetralogy of Fallot.
2. Third-degree heart block.

alt.: diagnoses, plural

OPERATION:
Pacemaker insertion, ventricular pacing, ventricular sensing, inhibited mode, epicardial, subrectus.

SURGEON:
XXXX

ANESTHESIA:
Given by pediatric intensivist.

INDICATIONS:
This 2-week-old girl was born with complex pulmonary atresia and tetralogy of Fallot, and underwent complete repair as a neonate. Postoperatively, the baby manifested sustained third-degree atrioventricular block and was pacing using the temporary leads placed intraoperatively. With absence of return of conduction after 1-1/2 weeks, a pacemaker is now justified.

PROCEDURE:
Following induction of anesthesia, the baby was sterilely prepped and draped and given IV antibiotics. A midline subxiphoid vertical incision was made and carried down into the left rectus sheath. The rectus muscle was reflected anteriorly and a plane developed between the posterior rectus sheath and rectus muscle to develop a generator packet. The incision was extended to the xiphoid process, then dissection carried out to the diaphragmatic edge and into the pericardial cavity; the inferior wall of the right ventricle was exposed. A steroid-eluding single 15-cm long epicardial lead was then fixated to the inferior wall of the right ventricle using two 5-0 Prolene mattress stitches. The lead was tested and had an R wave amplitude of 8.2 mV, with a pacing threshold of 0.9 V and an impedance of 439 ohms. The wound was thoroughly irrigated with antibiotic-saline solution. The lead was then

s/b pocket, typographical error

s/b eluting, common transcription error

(continued)

connected to a Medtronic Enpulse SR single-chamber generator, model #E2SR01, and the generator was placed in the pocket. After further antibiotic irritation, the temporary pacing leads were removed, given that there was good pacing using the generator. The wound was then closed in layers with running absorbable suture. In particular, the rectus sheath was reapproximated to the contralateral side very carefully to avoid epicardial hernia. Monofilament nylon was used to close the skin, and then a dry dressing was placed.

The baby tolerated the procedure apparently well. Care was continued after taking the baby back to the cardiac intensive care unit.

s/b irrigation, typographical error

For Signature

PACEMAKER INSERTION (PEDIATRIC)

PACEMAKER REPORT

PREOPERATIVE DIAGNOSES:
1. Status post repair of pulmonary atresia and tetralogy of Fallot.
2. Third-degree heart block.

POSTOPERATIVE DIAGNOSES:
1. Status post repair of pulmonary atresia and tetralogy of Fallot.
2. Third-degree heart block.

OPERATION:
Pacemaker insertion, ventricular pacing, ventricular sensing, inhibited mode, epicardial, subrectus.

SURGEON:
XXXX

ANESTHESIA:
Given by pediatric intensivist.

INDICATIONS:
This 2-week-old girl was born with complex pulmonary atresia and tetralogy of Fallot, and underwent complete repair as a neonate. Postoperatively, the baby manifested sustained third-degree atrioventricular block and was pacing using the temporary leads placed intraoperatively. With absence of return of conduction after 1-1/2 weeks, a pacemaker is now justified.

PROCEDURE:
Following induction of anesthesia, the baby was sterilely prepped and draped and given IV antibiotics. A midline subxiphoid vertical incision was made and carried down into the left rectus sheath. The rectus muscle was reflected anteriorly and a plane developed between the posterior rectus sheath and rectus muscle to develop a generator pocket. The incision was extended to the xiphoid process, then dissection carried out to the diaphragmatic edge and into the pericardial cavity; the inferior wall of the right ventricle was exposed. A steroid-eluting, single 15-cm long epicardial lead was then fixated to the inferior wall of the right ventricle using two 5-0 Prolene mattress stitches. The lead was tested and had an R wave amplitude of 8.2 mV, with a pacing threshold of 0.9 V and an impedance of 439 ohms. The wound was thoroughly irrigated with antibiotic-saline solution. The lead was then connected to a Medtronic Enpulse SR single-chamber generator, model #E2SR01, and the generator was placed in the pocket. After further antibiotic irrigation, the temporary pacing leads were removed, given that there was good pacing using the generator. The wound was then closed in layers with running absorbable suture. In particular, the rectus sheath was reapproximated to the contralateral side very carefully to avoid epicardial hernia. Monofilament nylon was used to close the skin, and then a dry dressing was placed.

The baby tolerated the procedure apparently well. Care was continued after taking the baby back to the cardiac intensive care unit.

Answer Key

TRANSCATHETER OCCLUSION OF PATENT FORAMEN OVALE

PERCUTANEOUS CORONARY INTERVENTION

PROCEDURE: Transcatheter occlusion of patent foramen ovale

PREPROCEDURE DIAGNOSIS: Patent foramen ovale

POSTPROCEDURE DIAGNOSIS: Patent foramen ovale

insert period, AAMT Book of Style, formats

INDICATIONS: This 64-year-old lady presented with a stroke ten days ago. This was confirmed to be an embolic event, with no other source identified. She was felt to be a poor candidate for anticoagulation therapy, and after discussion with her cardiologist and neurologist, we agreed to consider transcatheter occlusion of a patent foramen ovale. Detailed discussion was undertaken with patient and her hubby prior to embarking on the procedure, including the risks, benefits and alternatives to the use of device occlusion of the patent foramen ovale. Informed consent was obtained.

s/b husband, do not use slang terms

PROCEDURE DETAILS: Patient was sedated with Versed and fentanyl, as supervised by cardiac anesthesia. Xylocaine 2% local anesthesia was infiltrated into the right groin, after prepping and draping in the usual manner. Percutaneous entry into the right femoral vein was obtained and a 10-French sheath inserted. This allowed passage of a multipurpose catheter across the patent foramen ovale. Utilizing the multipurpose catheter, a 0.035-inch Amplatz wire was introduced from the right atrium to the left atrium, across the patent foramen ovale, and anchored in the left lower pulmonary vein. A 3-cm balloon seizing catheter was introduced across the patent foramen ovale. By fluoroscopy, the patent foramen ovale balloon sized to 9 mm.

s/b Cardiac Anesthesia, capitalize a department name that is referred to as an entity, AAMT Book of Style, business names, departments

s/b sizing, incorrect term

It should be noted that the patient was a poor candidate for general anesthesia, in view of the decreased ejection fraction; hence, she was not subjected to transesophageal echocardiography.

Utilizing fluoroscopy as a Marker, the short 10-French sheath was exchanged for a long 10-French sheath. An occlusion device was prepared in the usual manner and introduced via the 10-French sheath to the atrium. The distal left atrial portion of the device was delivered and, by fluoroscopy, confirmed to be against the

s/b marker, not capitalized because it is not a proper name, general rule of grammar

(continued)

left atrial side of the septum. Following this, the right atrial portion of the device was released as well. By fluoroscopy, the device was seen to be in excellent position. The device was released without complication. The 10-French sheath was exchanged for a short 10-French sheath, in order to allow for VasoSeal-assisted hemostasis. Catheters were removed, bleeding stopped by local pressure.

Patient was conscious and talking throughout the procedure and experienced no discomfort. The patient was transferred back to her floor for subsequent recovery.

Following the procedure, the patient will be maintained on aspirin 325 mg and Plavix 75 mg daily for a period of 6 months. Patient will have a chest x-ray as well as an echocardiogram 24 hours following the procedure and be maintained on 3 doses of Ancef over 24 hours.

For Signature

TRANSCATHETER OCCLUSION OF PATENT FORAMEN OVALE

PERCUTANEOUS CORONARY INTERVENTION

PROCEDURE: Transcatheter occlusion of patent foramen ovale.

PREPROCEDURE DIAGNOSIS: Patent foramen ovale.

POSTPROCEDURE DIAGNOSIS: Patent foramen ovale.

INDICATIONS: This 64-year-old lady presented with a stroke ten days ago. This was confirmed to be an embolic event, with no other source identified. She was felt to be a poor candidate for anticoagulation therapy, and after discussion with her cardiologist and neurologist, we agreed to consider transcatheter occlusion of a patent foramen ovale. Detailed discussion was undertaken with patient and her husband prior to embarking on the procedure, including the risks, benefits and alternatives to the use of device occlusion of the patent foramen ovale. Informed consent was obtained.

PROCEDURE DETAILS: Patient was sedated with Versed and fentanyl, as supervised by Cardiac Anesthesia. Xylocaine 2% local anesthesia was infiltrated into the right groin, after prepping and draping in the usual manner. Percutaneous entry into the right femoral vein was obtained and a 10-French sheath inserted. This allowed passage of a multipurpose catheter across the patent foramen ovale. Utilizing the multipurpose catheter, a 0.035-inch Amplatz wire was introduced from the right atrium to the left atrium, across the patent foramen ovale, and anchored in the left lower pulmonary vein. A 3-cm balloon sizing catheter was introduced across the patent foramen ovale. By fluoroscopy, the patent foramen ovale balloon sized to 9 mm.

It should be noted that the patient was a poor candidate for general anesthesia, in view of the decreased ejection fraction; hence, she was not subjected to transesophageal echocardiography.

Utilizing fluoroscopy as a marker, the short 10-French sheath was exchanged for a long 10-French sheath. An occlusion device was prepared in the usual manner and introduced via the 10-French sheath to the atrium. The distal left atrial portion of the device was delivered and, by fluoroscopy, confirmed to be against the left atrial side of the septum. Following this, the right atrial portion of the device was released as well. By fluoroscopy, the device was seen to be in excellent position. The device was released without complication. The 10-French sheath was exchanged for a short 10-French sheath, in order to allow for VasoSeal-assisted hemostasis. Catheters were removed, bleeding stopped by local pressure.

Patient was conscious and talking throughout the procedure and experienced no discomfort. The patient was transferred back to her floor for subsequent recovery.

Following the procedure, the patient will be maintained on aspirin 325 mg and Plavix 75 mg daily for a period of 6 months. Patient will have a chest x-ray as well as an echocardiogram 24 hours following the procedure and be maintained on 3 doses of Ancef over 24 hours.

Answer Key

ELECTROPHYSIOLOGIC STUDY

ELECTROPHYSIOLOGIC STUDY

PROCEDURE: Electrophysiologic study.

CLINICAL HISTORY: A very pleasant 75-year-old gentleman with ischemic heart disease, with syncopal episode associated with motor vehicle accident and severe trauma. Patient has undergone recent PCI. He is aware of the risks, benefits, and alternatives to proceeding with electrophysiologic study for further assessment.

He is aware that these risks include, but are not limited to, infection, death, stroke, myocardial infarction, vessel damage, limb damage, pain, pneumothorax, deep venous thrombosis, pulmonary embolus, need for vascular repair, need for transfusion, need for device and/or lead repoisoning, and the possibility that this might not improve, and even worsen, his situation. He understands and wishes to proceed with electrophysiologic study.

s/b repositioning, typographical error

PROCEDURE/TECHNIQUE: After informed consent was obtained, the patient was brought to the EP laboratory in a fasting state. He was prepped and draped in the usual sterile fashion with multiple layers of Betadine. Pilocaine 1% infiltration was used to achieve local anesthesia over the left inguinal area. Using a #18-gauge needle and a 0.035 guidewire, access was obtained into the left femoral vein. Over the guidewire, a 5-French sheath was advanced into this vessel. Using identical technique at 2 separate sites along the course of the left femoral vein, two 6-French sheaths were advanced. Through these sheaths, one 6-French and two 5-French, 5-mm quadripolar electrode catheters were advanced, using fluoroscopic and electrocardiographic guidance, to positions in the high right atrium, right ventricular apex, and to a position across the tricuspid annulus such that a Hiss bundle electrogram could be carefully mapped and recorded. After baseline intervals and pacing thresholds were obtained, RA and RV incremental pacing and programmed stimulation were performed. Sinus node recovery times were performed. Carotid sinus massage was performed. At the end of the procedure, all catheters and sheaths were removed. He tolerated the procedure quite well and returned to the recovery area in stable condition.

s/b Polocaine, common transcription error

s/b His, misspelled (pronounced like hiss), Stedman's Medical Dictionary, 28E

(continued)

FINDINGS:

1. At baseline, intracardiac intervals are normal, with an A-H interval of 90 msec and an H-V interval of 52 msec.
2. Markedly abnormal sinus node function is demonstrated. Corrected sinus node recovery times are reproducibly increased up to 3500 msec. This is a reproducible finding.
3. AV nodal function is normal with an antegrade AV nodal refractory period of 700/440 and an antegrade Wenckebach cycle length of 450 msec.
4. No supraventricular arrhythmias are inducible.
5. There is no evidence of an accessory bypass track. All conductions are central through the AV node in both the antegrade and retrograde directions; both antegrade and retrograde Wenckebach are seen.
6. No pathologic pauses or hypotension is noted with right-sided or left-sided carotid sinus massage.
7. Episodes of ventricular tachycardia are reproducibly inducible during drive cycle lengths of 400 msec, from both the right ventricular apex and the right ventricular outflow tract. These episodes are prolonged but self terminating.

s/b tract, Stedman's Medical Dictionary, 28E

s/b self-terminating, hyphenate compounds formed with the prefix self-, AAMT Book of Style, prefixes

CONCLUSION: This is a markedly abnormal electrophysiologic study with both ventricular tachycardia and evidence for sinus node dysfunction. Given the patient's ischemic myopathy, syncope with trauma, I will recommend a dual-chamber transvenous pectoral defibrillator.

For Signature

ELECTROPHYSIOLOGY STUDY

ELECTROPHYSIOLOGIC STUDY

PROCEDURE: Electrophysiologic study.

CLINICAL HISTORY: A very pleasant 75-year-old gentleman with ischemic heart disease, with syncopal episode associated with motor vehicle accident and severe trauma. Patient has undergone recent PCI. He is aware of the risks, benefits, and alternatives to proceeding with electrophysiologic study for further assessment.

He is aware that these risks include, but are not limited to, infection, death, stroke, myocardial infarction, vessel damage, limb damage, pain, pneumothorax, deep venous thrombosis, pulmonary embolus, need for vascular repair, need for transfusion, need for device and/or lead repositioning, and the possibility that this might not improve, and even worsen, his situation. He understands and wishes to proceed with electrophysiologic study.

PROCEDURE/TECHNIQUE: After informed consent was obtained, the patient was brought to the EP laboratory in a fasting state. He was prepped and draped in the usual sterile fashion with multiple layers of Betadine. Polocaine 1% infiltration was used to achieve local anesthesia over the left inguinal area. Using a #18-gauge needle and a 0.035 guidewire, access was obtained into the left femoral vein. Over the guidewire, a 5-French sheath was advanced into this vessel. Using identical technique at 2 separate sites along the course of the left femoral vein, two 6-French sheaths were advanced. Through these sheaths, one 6-French and two 5-French, 5-mm quadripolar electrode catheters were advanced, using fluoroscopic and electrocardiographic guidance, to positions in the high right atrium, right ventricular apex, and to a position across the tricuspid annulus such that a His bundle electrogram could be carefully mapped and recorded. After baseline intervals and pacing thresholds were obtained, RA and RV incremental pacing and programmed stimulation were performed. Sinus node recovery times were performed. Carotid sinus massage was performed. At the end of the procedure, all catheters and sheaths were removed. He tolerated the procedure quite well and returned to the recovery area in stable condition.

FINDINGS:
1. At baseline, intracardiac intervals are normal, with an A-H interval of 90 msec and an H-V interval of 52 msec.
2. Markedly abnormal sinus node function is demonstrated. Corrected sinus node recovery times are reproducibly increased up to 3500 msec. This is a reproducible finding.
3. AV nodal function is normal with an antegrade AV nodal refractory period of 700/440 and an antegrade Wenckebach cycle length of 450 msec.
4. No supraventricular arrhythmias are inducible.
5. There is no evidence of an accessory bypass tract. All conductions are central through the AV node in both the antegrade and retrograde directions; both antegrade and retrograde Wenckebach are seen.
6. No pathologic pauses or hypotension is noted with right-sided or left-sided carotid sinus massage.

(continued)

7. Episodes of ventricular tachycardia are reproducibly inducible during drive cycle lengths of 400 msec, from both the right ventricular apex and the right ventricular outflow tract. These episodes are prolonged but self-terminating.

CONCLUSION: This is a markedly abnormal electrophysiologic study with both ventricular tachycardia and evidence for sinus node dysfunction. Given the patient's ischemic myopathy, syncope with trauma, I will recommend a dual-chamber transvenous pectoral defibrillator.

Answer Key

ATRIOVENTRICULAR CANAL REPAIR WITH LIGATION OF PATENT DUCTUS ARTERIOSUS (PEDIATRIC)

OPERATIVE REPORT

PREOPERATIVE DIAGNOSES
1. Atrioventricular canal defect, transitional.
2. Ductus arteriosus.
3. Down syndrome.

POSTOPERATIVE DIAGNOSES
1. Atrioventricular canal defect, transitional.
2. Ductus arteriosus.
3. Down syndrome.

OPERATION
1. Atrioventricular canal defect repair, on cardiopulmonary bypass.
2. Ligation of ductus arteriosus.

SURGEON
XXXX

ASSISTANT
XXXX

ANESTHESIA
General.

INDICATIONS
This 7-month-old, 6-kg child with Down syndrome has a transitional atrioventricular canal defect. The child has been growing well, without overt failure. A recent follow-up echocardiogram revealed an atrioventricular canal defect with only a very small ventricular component to the shunt, with the septal crest largely covered over by accessory valve leaflet tissue. There was a moderate primum component to the canal, and a small patent foramen ovale. There was a cleft in the left atrioventricular valve, with minimal regurgitation.

s/b primam, misspelled

PROCEDURE
Following induction of anesthesia, the baby was sterilely prepped and draped and given IV antibiotics. A midline chest incision was made, carried down through the sternum with a saw, and a retractor placed. The thymus gland was excised and the pericardium was cleaned off, a patch excised and tanned in

(continued)

s/b *dissected*, incorrect term

s/b *mL*, ISMP List of Dangerous Abbreviations

s/b *were*, refers to *attachments*, plural

insert *bypass*, omitted word

s/b *ventricular-level*, insert hyphen; it's a shunt at the level of the ventricle, not a level shunt, AAMT Book of Style, compound modifiers

s/b *pledgeted*, misspelled, Stedman's Medical & Surgical Equipment Words, 4E

glutaraldehyde, and the remaining pericardium suspended on sutures. The ascending aorta and superior vena cava were resected out. The ductus arteriosus was exposed and ligated with a 2-0 Tevdek tie. Heparin 300 units/kg was given, bicaval cannulation completed, and cardiopulmonary begun with cooling to 28 degrees. Tourniquets were placed around the cavae, a vent was placed through the right superior pulmonary vein into the left ventricle, and a cardioplegic catheter placed. The aorta was occluded, and 25 cc/kg of crystalloid cardioplegia given, with maintenance doses of 10 cc/kg given every 20 to 30 minutes. The caval tourniquets were then tightened, an oblique right atriotomy made, and the edges suspended on traction stitches. The ventricles were suctioned of blood, then the canal defect was inspected. The primam defect was moderate, at most. We could not appreciate a ventricular component by direct but gentle probing. There was abundant attachments to the crest of the septum. Saline distention revealed a rather linear cleft between the superior and inferior bridging leaflets of the left AV valve, and a well-developed posterior leaflet. Though we could visualize the cleft through the primam defect, we could not readily expose it for closure. Therefore, we enlarged the primam defect by excising a small amount of septum from the superior lateral border of the defect. The left AV valve could now be much better visualized. The first marginal chords were located on the superior and inferior bridging leaflets, near the coaptation with the posterior leaflet. A 7-0 Prolene suture was then taken through the superior and inferior leaflets at this location and tied with three knots. One end was tagged, and this served to bring the valve up through the primam defect, where the cleft was now easily visualized. The cleft was then closed, running each arm of the 7-0 Prolene suture up to the septum. The cleft was not complete all the way to the septum, so we ran it to the sturdy accessory valve tissue at the base, near the septal attachments. The valve was then tested with saline distention and was completely competent, and had an adequate orifice. The small ventricular level shunt, if any, was probably at the location of the cleft near the crest of the septum. We closed this area with a pledgetted mattress suture of 6-0 Ethibond, and then tied this stitch to the Prolene cleft-closure stitch. The primam defect was then closed with the tanned pericardial patch and running 6-0 Prolene suture, with care taken to avoid the conduction system, as best as possible. The left atrium was distended with saline and the lungs ventilated to evacuate air prior to completion of this closure.

Rewarming was started. The patent foramen ovale was closed with a single mattress stitch of 6-0 Prolene. The right atrium was

(continued)

closed with doubly run 6-0 Prolene. After standard de-airing maneuvers, including an ascending aortic vent, the aortic clamp was removed, and the heart was reprofused. It began beating in spontaneous sinus rhythm during warming. The caval tourniquets were removed. Two right atrial catheters were placed and secured to the skin. A right ventricular pacing wire was placed and secured with a ground wire. Dopamine 5 mcg/kg per minute was started. With good cardiac activity, and after appropriate warming to 37 degrees core temperature, cardiopulmonary bypass was discontinued. Transesophageal echocardiography revealed no residual atrial or ventricular level shunts, and only trivial left AV valve and right AV valve regurgitation. The cannulas were thus removed, and protamine sulfate given. Hemostasis was rendered. The mediastinum was irrigated with antibiotic saline solution. The 16-French drain tube was placed and secured to the skin. After a final inspection and confirmation of counts, the chest was closed in layers with interrupted sternal wires and layers of running absorbable suture. An On-Q catheter was placed continuous Marcaine infusion. A dry dressing was placed. The baby tolerated the procedure apparently well, and care was continued in the cardiac ICU.

s/b reperfused, misspelled

insert *for* for clarity

For Signature

ATRIOVENTRICULAR CANAL REPAIR WITH LIGATION OF PATENT DUCTUS ARTERIOSUS (PEDIATRIC)

OPERATIVE REPORT

PREOPERATIVE DIAGNOSES
1. Atrioventricular canal defect, transitional.
2. Ductus arteriosus.
3. Down syndrome.

POSTOPERATIVE DIAGNOSES
1. Atrioventricular canal defect, transitional.
2. Ductus arteriosus.
3. Down syndrome.

OPERATION
1. Atrioventricular canal defect repair, on cardiopulmonary bypass.
2. Ligation of ductus arteriosus.

SURGEON
XXXX

ASSISTANT
XXXX

ANESTHESIA
General.

INDICATIONS
This 7-month-old, 6-kg child with Down syndrome has a transitional atrioventricular canal defect. The child has been growing well, without overt failure. A recent follow-up echocardiogram revealed an atrioventricular canal defect with only a very small ventricular component to the shunt, with the septal crest largely covered over by accessory valve leaflet tissue. There was a moderate primam component to the canal, and a small patent foramen ovale. There was a cleft in the left atrioventricular valve, with minimal regurgitation.

PROCEDURE
Following induction of anesthesia, the baby was sterilely prepped and draped and given IV antibiotics. A midline chest incision was made, carried down through the sternum with a saw, and a retractor placed. The thymus gland was excised and the pericardium was cleaned off, a patch excised and tanned in glutaraldehyde, and the remaining pericardium suspended on sutures. The ascending aorta and superior vena cava were dissected out. The ductus arteriosus was exposed and ligated with a 2-0 Tevdek tie. Heparin 300 units/kg was given, bicaval cannulation completed, and cardiopulmonary bypass begun with cooling to 28 degrees. Tourniquets were placed around the cavae, a vent was placed through the right superior pulmonary vein into the left ventricle, and a cardioplegic catheter placed. The aorta was occluded, and 25 mL/kg of crystalloid cardioplegia

(continued)

given, with maintenance doses of 10 mL/kg given every 20 to 30 minutes. The caval tourniquets were then tightened, an oblique right atriotomy made, and the edges suspended on traction stitches. The ventricles were suctioned of blood, then the canal defect was inspected. The primam defect was moderate, at most. We could not appreciate a ventricular component by direct but gentle probing. There were abundant attachments to the crest of the septum. Saline distention revealed a rather linear cleft between the superior and inferior bridging leaflets of the left AV valve, and a well-developed posterior leaflet. Though we could visualize the cleft through the primam defect, we could not readily expose it for closure. Therefore, we enlarged the primam defect by excising a small amount of septum from the superior lateral border of the defect. The left AV valve could now be much better visualized. The first marginal chords were located on the superior and inferior bridging leaflets, near the coaptation with the posterior leaflet. A 7-0 Prolene suture was then taken through the superior and inferior leaflets at this location and tied with three knots. One end was tagged, and this served to bring the valve up through the primam defect, where the cleft was now easily visualized. The cleft was then closed, running each arm of the 7-0 Prolene suture up to the septum. The cleft was not complete all the way to the septum, so we ran it to the sturdy accessory valve tissue at the base, near the septal attachments. The valve was then tested with saline distention and was completely competent, and had an adequate orifice. The small ventricular-level shunt, if any, was probably at the location of the cleft near the crest of the septum. We closed this area with a pledgeted mattress suture of 6-0 Ethibond, and then tied this stitch to the Prolene cleft-closure stitch. The primam defect was then closed with the tanned pericardial patch and running 6-0 Prolene suture, with care taken to avoid the conduction system, as best as possible. The left atrium was distended with saline and the lungs ventilated to evacuate air prior to completion of this closure.

Rewarming was started. The patent foramen ovale was closed with a single mattress stitch of 6-0 Prolene. The right atrium was closed with doubly run 6-0 Prolene. After standard de-airing maneuvers, including an ascending aortic vent, the aortic clamp was removed, and the heart was reperfused. It began beating in spontaneous sinus rhythm during warming. The caval tourniquets were removed. Two right atrial catheters were placed and secured to the skin. A right ventricular pacing wire was placed and secured with a ground wire. Dopamine 5 mcg/kg per minute was started. With good cardiac activity, and after appropriate warming to 37 degrees core temperature, cardiopulmonary bypass was discontinued. Transesophageal echocardiography revealed no residual atrial or ventricular level shunts, and only trivial left AV valve and right AV valve regurgitation. The cannulas were thus removed, and protamine sulfate given. Hemostasis was rendered. The mediastinum was irrigated with antibiotic saline solution. The 16-French drain tube was placed and secured to the skin. After a final inspection and confirmation of counts, the chest was closed in layers with interrupted sternal wires and layers of running absorbable suture. An On-Q catheter was placed for continuous Marcaine infusion. A dry dressing was placed. The baby tolerated the procedure apparently well, and care was continued in the cardiac ICU.

Answer Key

DUAL-CHAMBER AUTOMATIC IMPLANTABLE CARDIOVERTER DEFIBRILLATOR IMPLANTATION

CARDIOLOGY PROCEDURE REPORT

PROCEDURE: Dual-chamber defibrillator insertion.

INDICATIONS: Patient experiencing syncopal episodes, with significant conduction abnormalities as noted on a recent EP study. An AICD is expected to prevent these arrhythmias as well as prevent sudden cardiac death.

PROCEDURE/TECHNIQUE: After informed consent was obtained, the patient was brought to the electrophysiology laboratory. She was prepped and draped in surgical fashion. The right subclavian area was anesthetized with 1% Xylocaine. Using modified Seldinger technique, the right subclavian vein was cannulated twice, and guide wires were advanced to the level of the inferior vena cava and secured with hemostats. An area 1 inch inferior was anesthetized with 1% Xylocaine. Using a #15 scalpel, the skin was incised, and the incision was carried down to the prepectoral fascia using Bovie cautery. The prepectoral fascia was then split using scissors, and dissection was carried out inferiorly to create a pocket and superiorly to incorporate both wires into the wound. The first guide wire was then used to advance an 11-French tear-away sheath under fluoroscopic guidance into the left subclavian vein. The sheath was in turn used to advance a Medtronic ventricular lead, model #5706, serial #XXXX. This lead was advanced under fluoroscopic guidance to the level of the inferior vena cava. The sheath was torn away and pressure held over the puncture site until hemostasis was obtained. This lead was then fitted with a curved stylet and advanced into the right ventricular outflow tract. Using a straight stylet, the lead was slowly withdrawn until it advanced into the right ventricular apex. The active fixation helix was then deployed using the supplied tool. The lead was then tested and found to have R waves of 8.3 mV with a pacing threshold of 0.4 V at 0.5 msec pulse width and an impedance of 468 ohms. Ten-volt pacing did not elicit any diaphragmatic capture. These values were judged acceptable, so the lead was sutured into place with #0 silk and the supplied sleeve. The second guide wire was then used to advance a 7-French tear-away sheath under fluoroscopic guidance in the left subclavian vein. This sheath was in turn used to advance a Medtronic atrial lead, model #5706, serial #XXXX. This lead was

(continued)

---

guidewire and *guidewires* are also acceptable, Stedman's Medical Dictionary, 28E

s/b right, refer to body of report

advanced under fluoroscopic guidance to the level of the inferior vena cava. The sheath was torn away and pressure was held over the puncture site until hemostasis was obtained. The lead was then fitted with a J-shape stylet and advanced into the area of the right atrial appendage. With four clockwise turns of the lead body, the lead was actively fixed in place. The stylet was withdrawn, and the lead was tested and found to have P waves of 6.8 mV with a pacing threshold of 0.5 V at 1 msec pulse width and an impedance of 686 ohms. Ten-volt pacing did not elicit any phrenic nerve capture. These values were judged acceptable, so the lead was sutured in place with #0 silk and the supplied sleeve. The leads were then disconnected from the Pacing Systems Analyzer and connected to a Medtronic generator, model #4768, serial #XXXX. Each lead was identified by its markings and serial numbers and connected to the appropriate port, with the distal coil being connected to the high voltage negative pole. All connections were secured with a torque wrench. The device was then implanted into the newly created pocket, after a lavage with copious amounts of antibiotic-saline solution. The device was secured to the floor of the pocket using a #0 silk stitch. We then proceeded with device testing.

s/b high-voltage, insert hyphen, AAMT Book of Style, compound modifiers

Through the device, P waves were 6 mV and R waves were 8 mV. Pacing thresholds were 0.5 V at 0.5 msec in both channels. Atrial impedance was 680 ohms and ventricular impedance was 490 ohms. The patient was then heavily sedated with fentanyl and Versed. Using T-shock mode, sustained ventricular fibrillation was induced. This was quickly detected by the device, which charged and delivered a 28-joule biphasic countershock at an impedance of 900 ohms, successfully converting the rhythm to sinus. After waiting 10 minutes, sustained ventricular fibrillation was again induced. At this time, a 29-joule biphasic countershock was successful in converting the rhythm to sinus, at an impedance of 898 ohms. At this time, implant criteria was completed with defibrillation thresholds of less than or equal to 35 joules.

s/b were, plural, subject-verb agreement

The wound was closed using 2-0 Vicryl in interrupted sutures for the facial layer, 2-0 Vicryl in a running by-layer suture for the subcutaneous layer, and Indermil for the skin layer.

s/b fascial, typographical error

s/b bilayer, misspelled

The patient tolerated the procedure well without apparent complications and was transferred to Recovery in stable condition. A chest x-ray was ordered and is pending at the time of this dictation.

CONCLUSION: Successful implantation of transvenous dual chamber defibrillator, with defibrillator thresholds of less than or equal to 35 joules.

For Signature

DUAL-CHAMBER AUTOMATIC IMPLANTABLE CARDIOVERTER DEFIBRILLATOR IMPLANTATION

CARDIOLOGY PROCEDURE REPORT

PROCEDURE: Dual-chamber defibrillator insertion.

INDICATIONS: Patient experiencing syncopal episodes, with significant conduction abnormalities as noted on a recent EP study. An AICD is expected to prevent these arrhythmias as well as prevent sudden cardiac death.

PROCEDURE/TECHNIQUE: After informed consent was obtained, the patient was brought to the electrophysiology laboratory. She was prepped and draped in surgical fashion. The right subclavian area was anesthetized with 1% Xylocaine. Using modified Seldinger technique, the right subclavian vein was cannulated twice, and guidewires were advanced to the level of the inferior vena cava and secured with hemostats. An area 1 inch inferior was anesthetized with 1% Xylocaine. Using a #15 scalpel, the skin was incised, and the incision was carried down to the prepectoral fascia using Bovie cautery. The prepectoral fascia was then split using scissors, and dissection was carried out inferiorly to create a pocket and superiorly to incorporate both wires into the wound. The first guidewire was then used to advance an 11-French tear-away sheath under fluoroscopic guidance into the right subclavian vein. The sheath was in turn used to advance a Medtronic ventricular lead, model #5706, serial #XXXX. This lead was advanced under fluoroscopic guidance to the level of the inferior vena cava. The sheath was torn away and pressure held over the puncture site until hemostasis was obtained. This lead was then fitted with a curved stylet and advanced into the right ventricular outflow tract. Using a straight stylet, the lead was slowly withdrawn until it advanced into the right ventricular apex. The active fixation helix was then deployed using the supplied tool. The lead was then tested and found to have R waves of 8.3 mV with a pacing threshold of 0.4 V at 0.5 msec pulse width and an impedance of 468 ohms. Ten-volt pacing did not elicit any diaphragmatic capture. These values were judged acceptable, so the lead was sutured into place with #0 silk and the supplied sleeve. The second guidewire was then used to advance a 7-French tear-away sheath under fluoroscopic guidance in the right subclavian vein. This sheath was in turn used to advance a Medtronic atrial lead, model #5706, serial #XXXX. This lead was advanced under fluoroscopic guidance to the level of the inferior vena cava. The sheath was torn away and pressure was held over the puncture site until hemostasis was obtained. The lead was then fitted with a J-shape stylet and advanced into the area of the right atrial appendage. With four clockwise turns of the lead body, the lead was actively fixed in place. The stylet was withdrawn, and the lead was tested and found to have P waves of 6.8 mV with a pacing threshold of 0.5 V at 1 msec pulse width and an impedance of 686 ohms. Ten-volt pacing did not elicit any phrenic nerve capture. These values were judged acceptable, so the lead was sutured in place with #0 silk and the supplied sleeve. The leads were then disconnected from the Pacing Systems Analyzer and connected to a Medtronic generator, model #4768, serial #XXXX. Each lead was identified by its markings and serial numbers and connected to the appropriate port, with the distal coil being connected to the high-voltage negative pole. All connections were secured with a torque wrench. The device was then implanted into the

(continued)

newly created pocket, after a lavage with copious amounts of antibiotic-saline solution. The device was secured to the floor of the pocket using a #0 silk stitch. We then proceeded with device testing.

Through the device, P waves were 6 mV and R waves were 8 mV. Pacing thresholds were 0.5 V at 0.5 msec in both channels. Atrial impedance was 680 ohms and ventricular impedance was 490 ohms. The patient was then heavily sedated with fentanyl and Versed. Using T-shock mode, sustained ventricular fibrillation was induced. This was quickly detected by the device, which charged and delivered a 28-joule biphasic countershock at an impedance of 900 ohms, successfully converting the rhythm to sinus. After waiting 10 minutes, sustained ventricular fibrillation was again induced. At this time, a 29-joule biphasic countershock was successful in converting the rhythm to sinus, at an impedance of 898 ohms. At this time, implant criteria were completed with defibrillation thresholds of less than or equal to 35 joules.

The wound was closed using 2-0 Vicryl in interrupted sutures for the fascial layer, 2-0 Vicryl in a running bilayer suture for the subcutaneous layer, and Indermil for the skin layer.

The patient tolerated the procedure well without apparent complications and was transferred to Recovery in stable condition. A chest x-ray was ordered and is pending at the time of this dictation.

CONCLUSION: Successful implantation of transvenous dual chamber defibrillator, with defibrillator thresholds of less than or equal to 35 joules.

Answer Key

COMPLEX PERCUTANEOUS INTERVENTION ON PERIPHERAL VASCULATURE

PERIPHERAL INTERVENTION PROCEDURE

PROCEDURE:
1. Antegrade right popliteal artery FoxHollow arthrectomy and angiogram.
2. Antegrade right anterior tibial artery proximal and distal segment rotational arthrectomy with 1.5 and 2.5 mm burs, percutaneous transluminal angioplasty, and angiography.
3. Right proximal dorsalis pedis artery FoxHollow arthrectomy, percutaneous transluminal angioplasty, and angiography.
4. Antegrade left distal posterior tibial artery percutaneous transluminal angioplasty and angiography.

CLINICAL HISTORY:
Patient is a 73-year-old male with a nonhealing foot ulcer.

TECHNIQUE:
Consent was obtained after explaining the risks, benefits, and alternatives, risks involving renal failure, retroperitoneal hemorrhage, bleeding, stroke, distal embolization, and imponderables. With a single stick, access was gained into the right common femoral artery by antegrade technique. We crossed the subtotally occluded anterior tibial artery via a stiff glide wire, which we exchanged over a Quick-Cross catheter to a PT Graphix wire. This was exchanged over a Transit catheter to a RotaWire floppy guide. Nitroglycerin 200 mcg was given to defuse spasm. Angiomax was administered. This was followed by rotational arthrectomy of the anterior tibial artery with a 1.5 mm bur. Multiple cuts were made in the proximal, mid, and distal segments. This resulted in a reduction of stenosis to about 70%. This was followed by rotational arthrectomy with a 2.0 mm bur in the proximal, mid, and distal segments. This followed by angiogram which revealed slow reflow-no reflow phenomenon. At this time, we administered papaverine 60 mg intraarterially, and gave 200 mcg of nitroglycerin intraarterially. There was slow flow detected. ReoPro intraarterial was administered as well, and a drip started.

At this time, we redirected the wire into the posterior tibial artery. FoxHollow arthrectomy of the popliteal artery was performed. Multiple cuts were made with a large amount of plaque removed.

(continued)

---

s/b 1.5- and 2.5-mm burs, AAMT Book of Style, hyphens, suspensive hyphens

s/b right because the entire procedure is carried out in the right leg

s/b 1.5-mm bur, use a hyphen to join a number and a unit of measure when they are used as an adjective preceding a noun, AAMT Book of Style, units of measure

s/b 2.0-mm bur

s/b atherectomy throughout, common dictation/ transcription error, Stedman's Medical Dictionary, 28E s/b *2 x 30-mm Maverick balloon*, AAMT Book of Style, compound modifiers, numerals with words

s/b *2 x 30-mm Maverick balloon*

spell out *anterior tibial artery*; do not use abbreviations in the impression section of a report, AAMT Book of Style, abbreviations, acronyms, brief forms

Stenosis was reduced from 70% to less than 20%, with no evidence of any dissection or embolization.

This was followed by PTA of the distal posterior tibial artery with a 2 x 30 mm Maverick balloon. Three inflations were made for 60 and 90 seconds each. Stenosis was reduced from 99% to less than 20%. There was flow seen into the plantar arch; however, there was diffuse, severe disease which was left untouched.

At this time, the wire was again redirected into the dorsalis pedis artery. Rotational arthrectomy was performed. This was followed by PTA with a 2.5 x 30 mm Maverick balloon to 6 atmospheres for 90 seconds. Stenosis was reduced to less than 20%. There was no evidence of any dissection or embolization.

NOTE:
This was an extremely complicated, long, drawn-out procedure with good results.

IMPRESSION:
1. Successful FoxHollow arthrectomy of the right popliteal artery.
2. Successful rotational arthrectomy and percutaneous transluminal angioplasty of the ATA.
3. Successful rotational arthrectomy and percutaneous transluminal angioplasty of the proximal dorsalis pedis artery.
4. Successful percutaneous transluminal angioplasty of the left posterior tibial artery distal segment.

PLAN:
At this point, patient has much better flow in his foot, with his wound having its best chance for healing. If this does not heal, we may not have any more interventional options left.

s/b *atherectomy*, common dictation/transcription error, Stedman's Medical Dictionary, 28E

s/b *right* because the entire procedure is carried out in the right leg

For Signature

Report #29

COMPLEX PERCUTANEOUS INTERVENTION ON PERIPHERAL VASCULATURE

PERIPHERAL INTERVENTION PROCEDURE

PROCEDURE:
1. Antegrade right popliteal artery FoxHollow atherectomy and angiogram.
2. Antegrade right anterior tibial artery proximal and distal segment rotational atherectomy with 1.5- and 2.5-mm burs, percutaneous transluminal angioplasty, and angiography.
3. Right proximal dorsalis pedis artery FoxHollow atherectomy, percutaneous transluminal angioplasty, and angiography.
4. Antegrade right distal posterior tibial artery percutaneous transluminal angioplasty and angiography.

CLINICAL HISTORY:
Patient is a 73-year-old male with a nonhealing foot ulcer.

TECHNIQUE:
Consent was obtained after explaining the risks, benefits, and alternatives, risks involving renal failure, retroperitoneal hemorrhage, bleeding, stroke, distal embolization, and imponderables. With a single stick, access was gained into the right common femoral artery by antegrade technique. We crossed the subtotally occluded anterior tibial artery via a stiff glide wire, which we exchanged over a Quick-Cross catheter to a PT Graphix wire. This was exchanged over a Transit catheter to a RotaWire floppy guide. Nitroglycerin 200 mcg was given to defuse spasm. Angiomax was administered. This was followed by rotational atherectomy of the anterior tibial artery with a 1.5-mm bur. Multiple cuts were made in the proximal, mid, and distal segments. This resulted in a reduction of stenosis to about 70%. This was followed by rotational atherectomy with a 2.0-mm bur in the proximal, mid, and distal segments. This was followed by angiogram which revealed slow reflow-no reflow phenomenon. At this time, we administered papaverine 60 mg intraarterially, and gave 200 mcg of nitroglycerin intraarterially. There was slow flow detected. ReoPro intraarterial was administered as well, and a drip started.

At this time, we redirected the wire into the posterior tibial artery. FoxHollow atherectomy of the popliteal artery was performed. Multiple cuts were made with a large amount of plaque removed. Stenosis was reduced from 70% to less than 20%, with no evidence of any dissection or embolization.

This was followed by PTA of the distal posterior tibial artery with a 2 x 30-mm Maverick balloon. Three inflations were made for 60 and 90 seconds each. Stenosis was reduced from 99% to less than 20%. There was flow seen into the plantar arch; however, there was diffuse, severe disease which was left untouched.

At this time, the wire was again redirected into the dorsalis pedis artery. Rotational atherectomy was performed. This was followed by PTA with a 2.5 x 30-mm Maverick balloon to 6 atmospheres

(continued)

for 90 seconds. Stenosis was reduced to less than 20%. There was no evidence of any dissection or embolization.

NOTE:
This was an extremely complicated, long, drawn-out procedure with good results.

IMPRESSION:
1. Successful FoxHollow atherectomy of the right popliteal artery.
2. Successful rotational atherectomy and percutaneous transluminal angioplasty of the anterior tibial artery.
3. Successful rotational atherectomy and percutaneous transluminal angioplasty of the proximal dorsalis pedis artery.
4. Successful percutaneous transluminal angioplasty of the right posterior tibial artery distal segment.

PLAN:
At this point, patient has much better flow in his foot, with his wound having its best chance for healing. If this does not heal, we may not have any more interventional options left.

Answer Key

Report #30

CORRECTIVE SURGERY FOR COMPLEX CONGENITAL HEART DEFECTS (PEDIATRIC)

OPERATIVE REPORT

PREOPERATIVE DIAGNOSIS: D-transposition of the great arteries with large perimembranous ventricular septal defect and intramural right coronary artery, status post balloon atrial septostomy.

POSTOPERATIVE DIAGNOSIS: D-transposition of the great arteries with large perimembranous ventricular septal defect and intramural right coronary artery, status post balloon atrial septostomy.

OPERATION: Arterial switch procedure; ventricular septal defect closure using pericardial patch; atrial septal defect closure using pericardial patch; patent ductus arteriosus ligation and division.

SURGEON: XXXX

ASSISTANT: XXXX

ANESTHESIA: General.

INDICATIONS: This 5-day-old, 2200-gm boy was followed in fetal life with transposition of the great vessels and a ventricular septal defect. The baby was born at 37 weeks and was mildly cyanotic. Echocardiography revealed the above diagnosis. There was a large perimembranous ventricular septal defect. There was a right anterior aorta from which 2 coronary ostia could be seen. The right coronary, however, appeared to empty fairly high in the root, indicating an intramural course. The left gave rise to the circumflex in the anterior facing sinus. Balloon atrial septostomy was performed to stabilize the baby. The baby was then brought to the operating room a few days later for the following procedure.

PROCEDURE: Following induction of amnesia, the baby was sterilely prepped and draped and given IV antibiotics. A midline chest incision was made and carried down through the sternum, and a retractor placed. The thymus gland was incised. The pericardium was cleaned off and a generous patch excised and tanned in glutaraldehyde. Remaining pericardium was opened. The innominate vein was mobilized. Then, the great vessels, including the main pulmonary artery and both branches, were

(continued)

Margin notes:

write out *dextrotransposition*, diagnostic terms for preoperative and postoperative diagnosis should be spelled out, AAMT Book of Style, diagnosis

list names of operations vertically, AAMT Book of Style, formats

s/b anesthesia, incorrect term

s/b excised, common practice during pediatric cardiac surgery mobilized. The ductus arteriosus was exposed. A pantaloon patch of pulmonary homograft was sawed then trimmed appropriately. Marking sutures of 7-0 Prolene were placed on the matching sinuses for the proposed site of coronary artery transfer. The right coronary artery lacked an ostial bulge, but its intramural course was partially visible as a prominence that went 4 to 5 mm distal and posterior on the anterior root. Heparin, 300 units/kg, was given, then a straight venous cannula was placed in the atrium and angled in the inferior vena cava. An 8-French arterial cannula was placed. Cardiopulmonary bypass was begun with cooling to 18 degrees over 25 minutes. The ductus arteriosus was further dissected out, then ligated on the aortic side with a 2-0 Tevdek tie. A vent was placed through the right pulmonary vein into the left ventricle, tourniquets placed around the cavae; a point of proposed division of the anterior great artery was chosen, and a cardioplegic catheter was placed there. The aorta was occluded with a clamp, and 25 mL/kg of crystalloid cardioplegia was given, with subsequent doses of 10 mL/kg given every 20 to 30 minutes, using an olive-tipped catheter. The right atrial cannula was now advanced into the superior vena cava and secured with a tourniquet, and the inferior caval tourniquet was tightened. An oblique right atriotomy incision was made and traction sutures placed. Through the tricuspid valve, a large perimembranous defect could easily be seen. Traction sutures were placed on the septal leaf, on the anterior leaflet, and then a Tevdek tie placed around some prominent chords of the septal leaflet. With this exposure, the ventricular septal defect was now closed with a pericardial patch and running 7-0 Prolene suture. The tricuspid valve was tested and was competent. The atrial septal defect was large and there was foraminal tissue loss. Therefore, this was closed with a second pericardial patch and running 7-0 Prolene suture. The right atriotomy was then partially closed with running, doubly run 6-0 Prolene suture. A maintenance dose of cardioplegia was given, and the cardioplegic catheter was removed; the aorta was divided at that location. The route was inspected, and the entry point of the right coronary artery could be seen just above the posterior commissure and directly next to it. The left coronary ostium was separate in the anterior sinus, as expected. The ductus arteriosus was now doubly ligated with a 6-0 Prolene pursestring suture, then divided. Then, the main pulmonary artery was divided distal to the marking sutures, near its bifurcation. The branch pulmonary arteries were then completely mobilized with cautery and a LeCompte maneuver performed. A traction suture was placed on the anterior root to bring both roots anteriorly. The coronary ostia were again inspected, then generous buttons cut out, using

s/b thawed, incorrect term

s/b root, incorrect term

(continued)

tenotomy scissors. The right coronary artery required takedown of the posterior commissure of the anterior valve in order to achieve an adequate-size button. Both buttons were then mobilized with low-power cautery and care was taken to preserve all coronary artery branches possible. A U-shaped incision was then made in the matching sinuses, and root tissue was removed to achieve a better circumferential match with the aortic arch. Each coronary was then implanted into its matching location on the posterior root using running 7-0 Maxon suture. Each suture arm was tied to a separately placed 7-0 Maxon stitch. Aorta was then anastomosed to the posterior root using a running 7-0 Maxon suture. At near-completion, the olive-tipped catheter was placed in the aortic root and a dose of cardioplegia given in order to observe coronary filling and general anatomy. The coronaries filled nicely and the anatomy appeared appropriate. Now, the pantaloon pulmonary homograft patch was used to reconstruct the anterior root, resuspending the commissure to the homograft patch. The patch was then trimmed. The patient was placed in partial Trendelenburg and the heart allowed to fill some while de-airing through suture lines. The aortic clamp was then removed. Both coronary systems filled well and the heart began beating in spontaneous sinus rhythm. The pulmonary bifurcation was then anastomosed to the anterior root using a running 7-0 Prolene suture. The ductal tissue on the bifurcation area was extremely friable and de-hissed during placement of the bifurcation sutures. Therefore, in place of all ductal tissue, we replaced the superior portion of the bifurcation area with a separate patch of pulmonary homograft. This assured that both left and right pulmonary branches were wide open and under no tension. Rewarming was started. Suture lines were inspected for hemostasis. A single right atrial catheter was placed and secured to the skin. The pleural cavities were opened and drained of fluid. The caval tourniquets were removed. Milrinone, dopamine and epinephrine were started. The lungs were ventilated. There was good cardiac activity at 36 degrees core temperature and no evidence of coronary ischemia. There were no regional wall motion abnormalities as viewed directly. Cardiopulmonary bypass was then discontinued. The venous cannulas were removed. The hemodynamics were observed, and the right atrial pressure was 8 mmHg with a blood pressure of 65/30, a heart rate of 140 in sinus rhythm, with a narrow QRS complex. The QRS did seem to vary intermittently and suddenly, but with no hemodynamic compromise. There were no arrhythmias. The arterial cannula was therefore removed and protamine sulfate given. All suture lines were packed with thrombin-Gelfoam and Surgicel. Ultimately, good hemostasis was achieved. Surgical glue

s/b dehisced, misspelled

(continued)

was then applied to the suture lines. The mediastinum was thoroughly irrigated with antibiotic saline solution. A 16-French drain tube was placed, secured to the skin, and set to feeding tube suction. After a final inspection and confirmation of counts, the chest was closed in layers with interrupted stainless steel wires and layers of running absorbable suture. A dry dressing was placed. The baby tolerated the procedure apparently well, and care was continued in the cardiac intensive care unit.

For Signature

CORRECTIVE SURGERY FOR COMPLEX CONGENITAL HEART DEFECTS (PEDIATRIC)

OPERATIVE REPORT

PREOPERATIVE DIAGNOSIS: Dextrotransposition of the great arteries with large perimembranous ventricular septal defect and intramural right coronary artery, status post balloon atrial septostomy.

POSTOPERATIVE DIAGNOSIS: Dextrotransposition of the great arteries with large perimembranous ventricular septal defect and intramural right coronary artery, status post balloon atrial septostomy.

OPERATION:
Arterial switch procedure.
Ventricular septal defect closure using pericardial patch.
Atrial septal defect closure using pericardial patch.
Patent ductus arteriosus ligation and division.

SURGEON: XXXX

ASSISTANT: XXXX

ANESTHESIA: General.

INDICATIONS: This 5-day-old, 2200-gm boy was followed in fetal life with transposition of the great vessels and a ventricular septal defect. The baby was born at 37 weeks and was mildly cyanotic. Echocardiography revealed the above diagnosis. There was a large perimembranous ventricular septal defect. There was a right anterior aorta from which two coronary ostia could be seen. The right coronary, however, appeared to empty fairly high in the root, indicating an intramural course. The left gave rise to the circumflex in the anterior facing sinus. Balloon atrial septostomy was performed to stabilize the baby. The baby was then brought to the operating room a few days later for the following procedure.

PROCEDURE: Following induction of anesthesia, the baby was sterilely prepped and draped and given IV antibiotics. A midline chest incision was made and carried down through the sternum, and a retractor placed. The thymus gland was excised. The pericardium was cleaned off and a generous patch excised and tanned in glutaraldehyde. Remaining pericardium was opened. The innominate vein was mobilized. Then, the great vessels, including the main pulmonary artery and both branches, were mobilized. The ductus arteriosus was exposed. A pantaloon patch of pulmonary homograft was thawed then trimmed appropriately. Marking sutures of 7-0 Prolene were placed on the matching sinuses for the proposed site of coronary artery transfer. The right coronary artery lacked an ostial bulge, but its intramural course was partially visible as a prominence that went 4 to 5 mm distal and posterior on the anterior root. Heparin, 300 units/kg, was given, then a straight venous cannula was placed in the atrium and angled in the inferior vena cava. An 8-French arterial cannula was placed. Cardiopulmonary bypass was begun with cooling to 18 degrees over 25 minutes. The ductus arteriosus was further dissected out, then ligated on the aortic side with a 2-0 Tevdek tie. A vent was placed through the right pulmonary vein into the left

(continued)

ventricle, tourniquets placed around the cavae; a point of proposed division of the anterior great artery was chosen, and a cardioplegic catheter was placed there. The aorta was occluded with a clamp, and 25 mL/kg of crystalloid cardioplegia was given, with subsequent doses of 10 mL/kg given every 20 to 30 minutes, using an olive-tipped catheter. The right atrial cannula was now advanced into the superior vena cava and secured with a tourniquet, and the inferior caval tourniquet was tightened. An oblique right atriotomy incision was made and traction sutures placed. Through the tricuspid valve, a large perimembranous defect could easily be seen. Traction sutures were placed on the septal leaf, on the anterior leaflet, and then a Tevdek tie placed around some prominent chords of the septal leaflet. With this exposure, the ventricular septal defect was now closed with a pericardial patch and running 7-0 Prolene suture. The tricuspid valve was tested and was competent. The atrial septal defect was large and there was foraminal tissue loss. Therefore, this was closed with a second pericardial patch and running 7-0 Prolene suture. The right atriotomy was then partially closed with running, doubly run 6-0 Prolene suture. A maintenance dose of cardioplegia was given, and the cardioplegic catheter was removed; the aorta was divided at that location. The root was inspected, and the entry point of the right coronary artery could be seen just above the posterior commissure and directly next to it. The left coronary ostium was separate in the anterior sinus, as expected. The ductus arteriosus was now doubly ligated with a 6-0 Prolene pursestring suture, then divided. Then, the main pulmonary artery was divided distal to the marking sutures, near its bifurcation. The branch pulmonary arteries were then completely mobilized with cautery and a LeCompte maneuver performed. A traction suture was placed on the anterior root to bring both roots anteriorly. The coronary ostia were again inspected, then generous buttons cut out, using tenotomy scissors. The right coronary artery required takedown of the posterior commissure of the anterior valve in order to achieve an adequate-size button. Both buttons were then mobilized with low-power cautery and care was taken to preserve all coronary artery branches possible. A U-shaped incision was then made in the matching sinuses, and root tissue was removed to achieve a better circumferential match with the aortic arch. Each coronary was then implanted into its matching location on the posterior root using running 7-0 Maxon suture. Each suture arm was tied to a separately placed 7-0 Maxon stitch. Aorta was then anastomosed to the posterior root using a running 7-0 Maxon suture. At near-completion, the olive-tipped catheter was placed in the aortic root and a dose of cardioplegia given in order to observe coronary filling and general anatomy. The coronaries filled nicely and the anatomy appeared appropriate. Now, the pantaloon pulmonary homograft patch was used to reconstruct the anterior root, resuspending the commissure to the homograft patch. The patch was then trimmed. The patient was placed in partial Trendelenburg and the heart allowed to fill some while de-airing through suture lines. The aortic clamp was then removed. Both coronary systems filled well and the heart began beating in spontaneous sinus rhythm. The pulmonary bifurcation was then anastomosed to the anterior root using a running 7-0 Prolene suture. The ductal tissue on the bifurcation area was extremely friable and dehisced during placement of the bifurcation sutures. Therefore, in place of all ductal tissue, we replaced the superior portion of the bifurcation area with a separate patch of pulmonary homograft. This assured that both left and right pulmonary branches were wide open and under no tension. Rewarming was started. Suture lines were inspected for hemostasis. A single right atrial catheter was placed and secured to the skin. The pleural cavities were opened and drained of fluid. The caval tourniquets were removed. Milrinone, dopamine and epinephrine were started. The lungs were ventilated. There was good cardiac activity at 36 degrees core temperature and no evidence of coronary ischemia. There were no regional wall motion abnormalities as viewed directly. Cardiopulmonary bypass was then

(continued)

discontinued. The venous cannulas were removed. The hemodynamics were observed, and the right atrial pressure was 8 mmHg with a blood pressure of 65/30, a heart rate of 140 in sinus rhythm, with a narrow QRS complex. The QRS did seem to vary intermittently and suddenly, but with no hemodynamic compromise. There were no arrhythmias. The arterial cannula was therefore removed and protamine sulfate given. All suture lines were packed with thrombin-Gelfoam and Surgicel. Ultimately, good hemostasis was achieved. Surgical glue was then applied to the suture lines. The mediastinum was thoroughly irrigated with antibiotic saline solution. A 16-French drain tube was placed, secured to the skin, and set to feeding tube suction. After a final inspection and confirmation of counts, the chest was closed in layers with interrupted stainless steel wires and layers of running absorbable suture. A dry dressing was placed. The baby tolerated the procedure apparently well, and care was continued in the cardiac intensive care unit.

Answer Key

TWO-DIMENSIONAL STUDY

CARDIAC NONINVASIVE STUDY

PROCEDURE: Two-dimensional limited study.

INDICATION: This is a 64-year-old with a history of congestive heart failure. This test is being done to evaluate for interventricular dyssynchrony.

TECHNIQUE: This is a 2-D limited study. Ejection fraction appears to be 35%. In evaluating for intraventricular dyssynchrony, the septal to the posterior wall level of the papilla muscle is 120 msec, which is not significant. Tissue Doppler was done of the basil septal wall, basil inferior wall, basil anterior wall, basilar lateral wall. The QRS to the peak systolic velocity of the septal wall is 185 msec; the QRS to the peak systolic velocity of the inferior wall is 190 msec; the QRS to the peak systolic velocity of the anterior wall is 220 msec; the QRS to the peak systolic velocity of the lateral wall is 205 msec. This is not consistent with any significant of intraventricular dyssynchrony.

In evaluating for interventricular dyssynchrony, the aortic ejection delay is 75 msec, the pulmonic ejection delay is 120 msec. This is consistent with some degree of interventricular dyssynchrony.

CONCLUSION:
1. Moderate left ventricular dysfunction, estimated ejection fraction is 35%.
2. No evidence of interventricular dyssynchrony.
3. Evidence of some degree of intraventricular dyssynchrony.

s/b papillary, incorrect term

s/b basal, misspelled, Stedman's Medical Dictionary, 28E

delete *of,* unnecessary word

s/b intraventricular, incorrect term based on the text of the report

s/b interventricular, incorrect term based on the text of the report

For Signature

TWO-DIMENSIONAL STUDY

CARDIAC NONINVASIVE STUDY

PROCEDURE: Two-dimensional limited study.

INDICATION: This is a 64-year-old with a history of congestive heart failure. This test is being done to evaluate for interventricular dyssynchrony.

TECHNIQUE: This is a 2-D limited study. Ejection fraction appears to be 35%. In evaluating for intraventricular dyssynchrony, the septal to the posterior wall level of the papillary muscle is 120 msec, which is not significant. Tissue Doppler was done of the basal septal wall, basal inferior wall, basal anterior wall, basilar lateral wall. The QRS to the peak systolic velocity of the septal wall is 185 msec; the QRS to the peak systolic velocity of the inferior wall is 190 msec; the QRS to the peak systolic velocity of the anterior wall is 220 msec; the QRS to the peak systolic velocity of the lateral wall is 205 msec. This is not consistent with any significant intraventricular dyssynchrony.

In evaluating for interventricular dyssynchrony, the aortic ejection delay is 75 msec, the pulmonic ejection delay is 120 msec. This is consistent with some degree of interventricular dyssynchrony.

CONCLUSION:
1. Moderate left ventricular dysfunction, estimated ejection fraction is 35%.
2. No evidence of intraventricular dyssynchrony.
3. Evidence of some degree of interventricular dyssynchrony.

Answer Key

PERCUTANEOUS CORONARY INTERVENTION

OPERATIVE REPORT

PROCEDURE:
1. Placement of a guiding catheter in the right coronary artery.
2. Intravascular ultrasound of the right coronary artery.
3. Drug-eluting stent to the right coronary artery.

BRIEF HISTORY: A 71-year-old female with classic anginal symptoms, who underwent diagnostic catheterization preceding this intervention. There was a lesion of uncertain significance on a bend in the proximal right coronary artery, and we are asked to perform intervascular ultrasound and intervention, if needed.

s/b intravascular, typographical error

PROCEDURE SUMMARY: A 5-French sheath was exchanged for a 6-French sheath in the right femoral artery. Because of a history of a thrombocytopenia, a bolus of Angiomax was given. A 6-French JR4 guiding catheter with side holes was used to correlate the right coronary artery. Initial angiograms revealed a questionable 60% to 70% lesion on a bend after a conus branch, prior to the right ventricular branch. There was a second bend noted in this artery, felt to be less significant, after the right ventricular branch. A 0.014 Stabilizer wire was advanced distally, and spasm of the artery was noted with wire placement.

s/b cannulate, incorrect term

Subsequently, intravascular ultrasound was performed with several runs. There appeared to be a 70% to 80% inferior eccentric plaque noted at the area in question, in a very short discreet segment. Decision was then made to proceed with stenting.

s/b discrete, AAMT Book of Style, soundalikes

A 3 x 13-mm Cypher stent was then deployed at 14 atmospheres. This straightened out the bend and reduced the stenosis to 0%. There was some kinking noted at the end of the stent, at the site of the previously-described lesion, which improved with administration of intracoronary nitroglycerin.

delete hyphen; do not hyphenate modifying adverbs ending in ly, AAMT Book of Style, compound modifiers, adverb ending in -ly

The patient had no chest pain or EKG changes with deployment of the stent. She was started on Plavix at the end of the procedure and transferred to the recovery area.

SUMMARY: Intravascular ultrasound of the right coronary artery revealed a 70% eccentric short lesion, successfully stented with a 3 x 13 Cypher stent.

For Signature

Report #32

PERCUTANEOUS CORONARY INTERVENTION

OPERATIVE REPORT

PROCEDURE:
1. Placement of a guiding catheter in the right coronary artery.
2. Intravascular ultrasound of the right coronary artery.
3. Drug-eluting stent to the right coronary artery.

BRIEF HISTORY: A 71-year-old female with classic anginal symptoms, who underwent diagnostic catheterization preceding this intervention. There was a lesion of uncertain significance on a bend in the proximal right coronary artery, and we are asked to perform intravascular ultrasound and intervention, if needed.

PROCEDURE SUMMARY: A 5-French sheath was exchanged for a 6-French sheath in the right femoral artery. Because of a history of a thrombocytopenia, a bolus of Angiomax was given. A 6-French JR4 guiding catheter with side holes was used to cannulate the right coronary artery. Initial angiograms revealed a questionable 60% to 70% lesion on a bend after a conus branch, prior to the right ventricular branch. There was a second bend noted in this artery, felt to be less significant, after the right ventricular branch. A 0.014 Stabilizer wire was advanced distally, and spasm of the artery was noted with wire placement.

Subsequently, intravascular ultrasound was performed with several runs. There appeared to be a 70% to 80% inferior eccentric plaque noted at the area in question, in a very short discrete segment. Decision was then made to proceed with stenting.

A 3 x 13-mm Cypher stent was then deployed at 14 atmospheres. This straightened out the bend and reduced the stenosis to 0%. There was some kinking noted at the end of the stent, at the site of the previously described lesion, which improved with administration of intracoronary nitroglycerin.

The patient had no chest pain or EKG changes with deployment of the stent. She was started on Plavix at the end of the procedure and transferred to the recovery area.

SUMMARY: Intravascular ultrasound of the right coronary artery revealed a 70% eccentric short lesion, successfully stented with a 3 x 13 Cypher stent.

Answer Key

INTRACARDIAC ELECTROPHYSIOLOGIC STUDY AND RADIOFREQUENCY CATHETER ABLATION (PEDIATRIC)

ELECTROPHYSIOLOGY REPORT

PROCEDURE: Intracardiac electrophysiologic study and radiofrequency catheter ablation.

INDICATIONS: The patient is a 14-year-old with a history of recurrent SVT. She was referred for electrophysiologic study with the plan for catheter ablation.

PROCEDURE/TECHNIQUE: The patient was brought to the catheterization laboratory and prepped and draped in the usual sterile fashion. She was sedated and intubated by Cardiac Anesthesia. Access was obtained with 5-French and 8-French sheaths in the right femoral vein, two 5-French sheaths in the left femoral vein, and a 6-French sheath in the right internal jugular vein. A 5000-unit bolus of heparin was administered. ACT was monitored on an hourly basis. A 5-French quadripolar catheter was placed in the high right atrial appendage, a 5-French quadripolar catheter was placed in the right ventricular apex, and a 5-French Hisser catheter was placed in the anterior tricuspid groove to record a His bundle electrogram. A 5-French decapolar CS catheter was placed in the coronary sinus to record left-sided electrograms. Mapping and ablation were performed using a Bard D-curved ablation catheter. Baseline measurements were obtained. Atrial and ventricular stimulations were performed. A slow pathway ablation was performed. Repeat atrial and ventricular stimulations were performed. All catheters and sheaths were removed and hemostasis was obtained with Safeguard occlusion device. The patient was transported to the pediatric intensive care unit.

ELECTROPHYSIOLOGIC FINDINGS:

BASELINE MEASUREMENTS: Baseline recording demonstrated sinus rhythm at a cycle length of 629 msec. The A-H interval was 52, with an H-V interval of 42.

ATRIAL PACING: Atrial extrastimuli was placed in a drive train of 500 msec. There was evidence for dual AV node physiology with an A-H jump at 280 msec. Atrial ERP was 500/200. AV node ERP was not encountered. There were no AV node echo beats in the baseline state. Rapid atrial pacing demonstrated AV Wenckebach

s/b were, refers to stimuli, plural

(continued)

at 340 msec. Once again, there were no AV node echo beats or inducible SVT in the baseline state. Later in the case, following ventricular pacing, repeat atrial extrastimulus pacing and rapid atrial pacing were performed during Isuprel infusion and Isuprel elimination. During Isuprel elimination, the patient had reproducibly inducible SVT. The SVT had a cycle length of 289 msec with concentric activation in a VA of 18 msec, consistent with AV node reentry tachycardia. This was terminated with burst atrial pacing and, once again, reproducible.

s/b AVA, abbreviation for atrio-ventricular activation

VENTRICULAR PACING: Ventricular extrastimuli were placed in a drive train of 500 msec. There was concentric, decremental VA conduction. V ERP was 500/220. VA ERP was not encountered. Rapid ventricular pacing demonstrated VA block at 300 msec. There was no inducible SVT with ventricular pacing protocol. This protocol was repeated during an Isuprel infusion. Once again, there was no inducible SVT.

MAPPING AND ABLATION: Based on electrophysiologic findings, the patient was noted to have SVT due to AV node reentry tachycardia. Therefore, a slow pathway ablation was performed. The ablation catheter was positioned in the posteroseptal space, superior to the os of the coronary sinus. Of note, the coronary sinus so was quite dilated and the positioning was almost toward the mid-septal region. Application of radiofrequency energy was administered while there was a small atrial electrogram and a large ventricular electrogram. Initially, there was junctional acceleration where the atrial signals preceded the ventricular signals. The peak temperature during this lesion was approximately 54 degrees. The catheter was repositioned somewhat more superiorly. Repeat radiofrequency energy was administered for a total of 40 seconds, with a peak temperature of 56 degrees. During this time, there was junctional acceleration with 1:1 VA conduction.

s/b os, typographical error

POSTABLATION TESTING: Following slow pathway ablation, the patient was in sinus rhythm with normal AV conduction. Atrial extrastimulus pacing and rapid atrial pacing were performed in the baseline state, during Isuprel infusion, and during Isuprel elimination. This was repeated with two cycles of Isuprel infusion and Isuprel elimination, with repeat testing. The maximum response with very rapid atrial pacing was a single echo beat, with no inducible SVT.

IMPRESSION: Supraventricular tachycardia due to atrioventricular node reentry tachycardia. Acutely successful slow pathway ablation.

PLAN: The patient will be monitored in the pediatric intensive care unit. She will undergo an ECG and echocardiogram. Followup will be with her routine cardiologist in approximately 2 weeks.

For Signature

INTRACARDIAC ELECTROPHYSIOLOGIC STUDY AND RADIOFREQUENCY CATHETER ABLATION (PEDIATRIC)

ELECTROPHYSIOLOGY REPORT

PROCEDURE: Intracardiac electrophysiologic study and radiofrequency catheter ablation.

INDICATIONS: The patient is a 14-year-old with a history of recurrent SVT. She was referred for electrophysiologic study with the plan for catheter ablation.

PROCEDURE/TECHNIQUE: The patient was brought to the catheterization laboratory and prepped and draped in the usual sterile fashion. She was sedated and intubated by Cardiac Anesthesia. Access was obtained with 5-French and 8-French sheaths in the right femoral vein, two 5-French sheaths in the left femoral vein, and a 6-French sheath in the right internal jugular vein. A 5000-unit bolus of heparin was administered. ACT was monitored on an hourly basis. A 5-French quadripolar catheter was placed in the high right atrial appendage, a 5-French quadripolar catheter was placed in the right ventricular apex, and a 5-French Hisser catheter was placed in the anterior tricuspid groove to record a His bundle electrogram. A 5-French decapolar CS catheter was placed in the coronary sinus to record left-sided electrograms. Mapping and ablation were performed using a Bard D-curved ablation catheter. Baseline measurements were obtained. Atrial and ventricular stimulations were performed. A slow pathway ablation was performed. Repeat atrial and ventricular stimulations were performed. All catheters and sheaths were removed and hemostasis was obtained with Safeguard occlusion device. The patient was transported to the pediatric intensive care unit.

ELECTROPHYSIOLOGIC FINDINGS:

BASELINE MEASUREMENTS: Baseline recording demonstrated sinus rhythm at a cycle length of 629 msec. The A-H interval was 52, with an H-V interval of 42.

ATRIAL PACING: Atrial extrastimuli were placed in a drive train of 500 msec. There was evidence for dual AV node physiology with an A-H jump at 280 msec. Atrial ERP was 500/200. AV node ERP was not encountered. There were no AV node echo beats in the baseline state. Rapid atrial pacing demonstrated AV Wenckebach at 340 msec. Once again, there were no AV node echo beats or inducible SVT in the baseline state. Later in the case, following ventricular pacing, repeat atrial extrastimulus pacing and rapid atrial pacing were performed during Isuprel infusion and Isuprel elimination. During Isuprel elimination, the patient had reproducibly inducible SVT. The SVT had a cycle length of 289 msec with concentric activation in AVA of 18 msec, consistent with AV node reentry tachycardia. This was terminated with burst atrial pacing and, once again, reproducible.

VENTRICULAR PACING: Ventricular extrastimuli were placed in a drive train of 500 msec. There was concentric, decremental VA conduction. V ERP was 500/220. VA ERP was not encountered. Rapid ventricular pacing demonstrated VA block at 300 msec. There was no inducible SVT with ventricular pacing protocol. This protocol was repeated during an Isuprel infusion. Once again, there was no inducible SVT.

(continued)

MAPPING AND ABLATION: Based on electrophysiologic findings, the patient was noted to have SVT due to AV node reentry tachycardia. Therefore, a slow pathway ablation was performed. The ablation catheter was positioned in the posteroseptal space, superior to the os of the coronary sinus. Of note, the coronary sinus os was quite dilated and the positioning was almost toward the mid-septal region. Application of radiofrequency energy was administered while there was a small atrial electrogram and a large ventricular electrogram. Initially, there was junctional acceleration where the atrial signals preceded the ventricular signals. The peak temperature during this lesion was approximately 54 degrees. The catheter was repositioned somewhat more superiorly. Repeat radiofrequency energy was administered for a total of 40 seconds, with a peak temperature of 56 degrees. During this time, there was junctional acceleration with 1:1 VA conduction.

POSTABLATION TESTING: Following slow pathway ablation, the patient was in sinus rhythm with normal AV conduction. Atrial extrastimulus pacing and rapid atrial pacing were performed in the baseline state, during Isuprel infusion, and during Isuprel elimination. This was repeated with two cycles of Isuprel infusion and Isuprel elimination, with repeat testing. The maximum response with very rapid atrial pacing was a single echo beat, with no inducible SVT.

IMPRESSION: Supraventricular tachycardia due to atrioventricular node reentry tachycardia. Acutely successful slow pathway ablation.

PLAN: The patient will be monitored in the pediatric intensive care unit. She will undergo an ECG and echocardiogram. Followup will be with her routine cardiologist in approximately 2 weeks.

Answer Key

TRANSESOPHAGEAL ECHOCARDIOGRAM

CARDIOLOGY PROCEDURE REPORT

PROCEDURE: Transesophageal electrocardiogram.

INDICATIONS: An 81-year-old with weakness of the legs; study is ordered to evaluate for source of embolus.

s/b echocardiogram, incorrect term

TECHNIQUE: The transesophageal echocardiogram was performed without difficulty. Sedation was given in the form of 1 mg of Versed and 12.5 mg Demerol; the patient was adequately sedated with these dosages. Following probe placement, the overall LV function was evaluated and was 65%. There was evidence of a trace effusion noted. The aortic valve appeared to be trileaflet and slightly sclerotic, with Lamb excrescences seen, with trace aortic regurgitation noted. The mitral valve appeared to be apparently normal, with no mitral regurgitation. Trace tricuspid insufficiency was noted, with normal tricuspid valve. The pulmonary valve was well visualized and appeared to have mild pulmonic insufficiency. There was mild plaque seen of the aortic root. There was no evidence of ASD or VSD. The atrial appendage was well visualized and had no apparent clot.

s/b Lambl, misspelled, Stedman's Medical Dictionary, 28E

CONCLUSION: Preserved left ventricular function. Slight sclerosis of the aortic valve, with trace aortic insufficiency seen. There appears to be trace pericardial effusion. Mild pulmonic insufficiency is seen. Aortic valve has Lamb excrescences. In the ascending portion, there was some mild plaque seen in the aortic root, but there did not appear to be any thrombogenic material that would suggest a source of embolus. Overall ejection fraction was 60%.

For Signature

TRANSESOPHAGEAL ECHOCARDIOGRAM

CARDIOLOGY PROCEDURE REPORT

PROCEDURE: Transesophageal echocardiogram.

INDICATIONS: An 81-year-old with weakness of the legs; study is ordered to evaluate for source of embolus.

TECHNIQUE: The transesophageal echocardiogram was performed without difficulty. Sedation was given in the form of 1 mg of Versed and 12.5 mg Demerol; the patient was adequately sedated with these dosages. Following probe placement, the overall LV function was evaluated and was 65%. There was evidence of a trace effusion noted. The aortic valve appeared to be trileaflet and slightly sclerotic, with Lambl excrescences seen, with trace aortic regurgitation noted. The mitral valve appeared to be apparently normal, with no mitral regurgitation. Trace tricuspid insufficiency was noted, with normal tricuspid valve. The pulmonary valve was well visualized and appeared to have mild pulmonic insufficiency. There was mild plaque seen of the aortic root. There was no evidence of ASD or VSD. The atrial appendage was well visualized and had no apparent clot.

CONCLUSION: Preserved left ventricular function. Slight sclerosis of the aortic valve, with trace aortic insufficiency seen. There appears to be trace pericardial effusion. Mild pulmonic insufficiency is seen. Aortic valve has Lambl excrescences. In the ascending portion, there was some mild plaque seen in the aortic root, but there did not appear to be any thrombogenic material that would suggest a source of embolus. Overall ejection fraction was 60%.

Answer Key

LOWER EXTREMITY GRAFT IMAGING STUDY

VASCULAR IMAGING STUDY

TEST PERFORMED:
Lower extremity graft imaging study.

INDICATIONS:
The patient is a 61-year-old man with a right-to-left femorofemoral crossover graft and a left femoral-posterior tibial bypass graft, using composite arm veins. This is a surveying study.

Imaging of the left leg shows a widely patent graft down to just above the distal anastomosis where there is a velocity acceleration of 590 cm/second.

IMPRESSION:
Widely patient left femoral-posterior tibial bypass except for a high-grade stenosis of the graft just above the distal anastomosis.

s/b surveillance, incorrect term

s/b patent, typographical error

For Signature

LOWER EXTREMITY GRAFT IMAGING STUDY

VASCULAR IMAGING STUDY

TEST PERFORMED:
Lower extremity graft imaging study.

INDICATIONS:
The patient is a 61-year-old man with a right-to-left femorofemoral crossover graft and a left femoral-posterior tibial bypass graft, using composite arm veins. This is a surveillance study.

Imaging of the left leg shows a widely patent graft down to just above the distal anastomosis where there is a velocity acceleration of 590 cm/second.

IMPRESSION:
Widely patent left femoral-posterior tibial bypass except for a high-grade stenosis of the graft just above the distal anastomosis.

Answer Key

RIGHT GROIN IMAGING STUDY

VASCULAR IMAGING STUDY

STUDY TITLE
Right groin imaging study.

INDICATIONS
The patient is a 22-year-old man status post shotgun wound to the lateral aspect of the right thigh. This is a follow-up study of the right common femoral artery and vein.

STUDY
Imaging of the right medial thigh shows no evidence of an arterial or venous false aneurysm or fistula. There is no evidence of a deep venous thrombosis in the veins. Multiple shotgun pellets are seen.

IMPRESSION
There does not appear to be any injury to the arteries or veins in this area, nor any evidence of a venous thrombosis.

delete *study*, redundant

delete *in the veins*, redundant

For Signature

RIGHT GROIN IMAGING STUDY

VASCULAR IMAGING STUDY

STUDY TITLE
Right groin imaging.

INDICATIONS
The patient is a 22-year-old man status post shotgun wound to the lateral aspect of the right thigh. This is a follow-up study of the right common femoral artery and vein.

STUDY
Imaging of the right medial thigh shows no evidence of an arterial or venous false aneurysm or fistula. There is no evidence of a deep venous thrombosis. Multiple shotgun pellets are seen.

IMPRESSION
There does not appear to be any injury to the arteries or veins in this area, nor any evidence of a venous thrombosis.

Answer Key

PACEMAKER GENERATOR REPLACEMENT

PACEMAKER REPORT

PROCEDURE IN DETAIL: The patient was prepped in the usual sterile fashion. The right previous pacer site was in the right subclavian area. An incision was made. The pulse generator was removed. The ventricular lead was checked. Sensitivity was 5.8 mV, voltage 1.3 V, 2.4 mA, resistance 450 ohms. The same pacemaker pocket was used. A pulse generator (Affinity SR, serial number XXXXXX) was placed. The patient was sutured in the usual sterile fashion. The patient tolerated the procedure well.

use number symbol (#) for the word *number*, AAMT Book of Style Electronic, equipment terms

For Signature

PACEMAKER GENERATOR REPLACEMENT

PACEMAKER REPORT

PROCEDURE IN DETAIL: The patient was prepped in the usual sterile fashion. The right previous pacer site was in the right subclavian area. An incision was made. The pulse generator was removed. The ventricular lead was checked. Sensitivity was 5.8 mV, voltage 1.3 V, 2.4 mA, resistance 450 ohms. The same pacemaker pocket was used. A pulse generator (Affinity SR, serial #XXXXXX) was placed. The patient was sutured in the usual sterile fashion. The patient tolerated the procedure well.

Answer Key

Report #38

ELECTRICAL CARDIOVERSION

CARDIOLOGY PROCEDURE REPORT

PROCEDURE: Electrical cardioversion.

INDICATIONS: A 70-year-old, status post aortic valve replacement, thoracic aortic aneurysm repair with aortic valve conduct, and reimplantation of the coronary arteries, postoperatively has developed episodes of atrial fibrillation, atrial flutter, and atrial tachycardia.

s/b conduit, typographical error

On preconversion electrocardiogram, the patient's rhythm showed what may be in ectopic atrial tachycardia with a ventricular rate of 100 beats per minute, with a right bundle branch block pattern. We proceeded to perform synchronized electrical cardioversion.

s/b an, incorrect term

SEDATION: Versed 2 mg and 30 mg of Diprivan.

TECHNIQUE: Once adequate sedation was obtained, synchronized electrical cardioversion was performed with 20 jewels.

s/b joules or *J,* misspelled, Stedman's Medical Dictionary, 28E

Postconversion electrocardiogram shows well-defined atrial wave which is probably a sinus wave, with marked first-degree AV block. The other possibility is that this is a low atrial rhythm, end-conducted with first degree AV block. Flutter P waves are not identified.

The patient tolerated the procedure well.

For Signature

ELECTRICAL CARDIOVERSION

CARDIOLOGY PROCEDURE REPORT

PROCEDURE: Electrical cardioversion.

INDICATIONS: A 70-year-old, status post aortic valve replacement, thoracic aortic aneurysm repair with aortic valve conduit, and reimplantation of the coronary arteries, postoperatively has developed episodes of atrial fibrillation, atrial flutter, and atrial tachycardia.

On preconversion electrocardiogram, the patient's rhythm showed what may be an ectopic atrial tachycardia with a ventricular rate of 100 beats per minute, with a right bundle branch block pattern. We proceeded to perform synchronized electrical cardioversion.

SEDATION: Versed 2 mg and 30 mg of Diprivan.

TECHNIQUE: Once adequate sedation was obtained, synchronized electrical cardioversion was performed with 20 joules.

Postconversion electrocardiogram shows well-defined atrial wave which is probably a sinus wave, with marked first-degree AV block. The other possibility is that this is a low atrial rhythm, end-conducted with first degree AV block. Flutter P waves are not identified.

The patient tolerated the procedure well.

Answer Key

M-MODE, TWO-DIMENSIONAL ECHOCARDIOGRAM WITH COLOR FLOW DOPPLER

ECHOCARDIOGRAM

PROCEDURE: M-mode, two dimensional echocardiogram with color flow Doppler.

insert hyphen, s/b two-dimensional, AAMT Book of Style, hyphens, adjectives

INDICATION: Cardiac mass.

Left atrial cavity is mildly dilated, measuring approximately 4.2 cm. Mitral annular valve is mildly calcified. The aortic root is normal. The aortic valve leaflets are normal with normal leaflet extrusion. Ventricular cavity is mildly dilated, with global hypokinesia, and overall ejection fraction measuring 25%. There is a mobile mass present at the apex of the heart which appears to be a thrombus. This mass measures approximately 7 mm. The right atrium and right ventricular cavity are mildly dilated. No pericardial effusion is present. Doppler shows the presence of mild mitral and tricuspid regurgitation.

s/b excursion, incorrect term

CONCLUSION:
1. Cardiomyopathy with reduced ejection fraction of 25%.
2. Apical thrombus measuring 7 mm.
3. Mild mitral regurgitation.
4. Mild tricuspid regurgitation.
5. No pericardial effusion.

For Signature

M-MODE, TWO-DIMENSIONAL ECHOCARDIOGRAM WITH COLOR FLOW DOPPLER

ECHOCARDIOGRAM

PROCEDURE: M-mode, two-dimensional echocardiogram with color flow Doppler.

INDICATION: Cardiac mass.

Left atrial cavity is mildly dilated, measuring approximately 4.2 cm. Mitral annular valve is mildly calcified. The aortic root is normal. The aortic valve leaflets are normal with normal leaflet excursion. Ventricular cavity is mildly dilated, with global hypokinesia, and overall ejection fraction measuring 25%. There is a mobile mass present at the apex of the heart which appears to be a thrombus. This mass measures approximately 7 mm. The right atrium and right ventricular cavity are mildly dilated. No pericardial effusion is present. Doppler shows the presence of mild mitral and tricuspid regurgitation.

CONCLUSION:
1. Cardiomyopathy with reduced ejection fraction of 25%.
2. Apical thrombus measuring 7 mm.
3. Mild mitral regurgitation.
4. Mild tricuspid regurgitation.
5. No pericardial effusion.

Answer Key

ECHOCARDIOGRAM

ECHOCARDIOGRAM STUDY

FINDINGS:

1. Technically adequate study. Rhythm is irregular.
2. The echocardiographic appearance of the aortic valve is a normal-appearing semilunar valve with adequate excursion. There is mild aortic root sclerosis. The aortic root is of normal dimension. Mitral valve is mildly thickened with mildly decreased opening felt secondary to low cardiac output. Tricuspid and pulmonic valves was suboptimally imaged but appeared grossly normal.
3. Left atrium is moderately enlarged. Left ventricle is moderately dilated as well. Right atrium and right ventricle appear to be at upper limits of normal in dimensions.
4. The left ventricular wall thickness appears to be at upper limits of normal. The basal inferior segment is akinetic. Overall left ventricular contractility is moderately to severely impaired, with the ejection fraction estimated at 20% to 25%. Right ventricular contractility is moderately impaired.
5. No intracavitary mass, thrombus or valvular vegetations are identified.
6. No pericardial effusion is present.
7. Doppler reveals mild mitral regurgitation. There is increased E:A ratio, consistent with a restricted pattern of diastolic dysfunction. There is mild tricuspid regurgitation also present.

CONCLUSIONS:

1. Dilated cardiomyopathy with mildly dilated left ventricle and moderately dilated left atrium present. Severe global wall motion abnormalities as described above with severely impaired left ventricular systolic function. Impaired right ventricular function is also seen.
2. Fibrocalsific changes of the aortic and mitral valve without significant valvular disease.
3. Mild mitral and tricuspid regurgitation.

s/b were, AAMT Book of Style, subject-verb agreement

misspelled, s/b fibrocalcific, Stedman's Medical Dictionary, 28E

s/b valves

For Signature

Report #40

ECHOCARDIOGRAM

ECHOCARDIOGRAM STUDY

FINDINGS:

1. Technically adequate study. Rhythm is irregular.

2. The echocardiographic appearance of the aortic valve is a normal-appearing semilunar valve with adequate excursion. There is mild aortic root sclerosis. The aortic root is of normal dimension. Mitral valve is mildly thickened with mildly decreased opening felt secondary to low cardiac output. Tricuspid and pulmonic valves were suboptimally imaged but appeared grossly normal.

3. Left atrium is moderately enlarged. Left ventricle is moderately dilated as well. Right atrium and right ventricle appear to be at upper limits of normal in dimension.

4. The left ventricular wall thickness appears to be at upper limits of normal. The basal inferior segment is akinetic. Overall left ventricular contractility is moderately to severely impaired, with the ejection fraction estimated at 20% to 25%. Right ventricular contractility is moderately impaired.

5. No intracavitary mass, thrombus or valvular vegetations are identified.

6. No pericardial effusion is present.

7. Doppler reveals mild mitral regurgitation. There is increased E:A ratio consistent with a restricted pattern of diastolic dysfunction. There is mild tricuspid regurgitation also present.

CONCLUSIONS:

1. Dilated cardiomyopathy with mildly dilated left ventricle and moderately dilated left atrium present. Severe global wall motion abnormalities as described above with severely impaired left ventricular systolic function. Impaired right ventricular function is also seen.

2. Fibrocalcific changes of the aortic and mitral valve without significant valvular disease.

3. Mild mitral and tricuspid regurgitations.

Answer Key

ABNORMAL ELECTROPHYSIOLOGIC STUDY

ELECTROPHYSIOLOGIC STUDY

PROCEDURE:

Electrophysiologic study.

CLINICAL HISTORY:

Syncope.

PROCEDURE/TECHNIQUE:

After informed consent was obtained, the patient was brought to the laboratory in a fasting state. He was prepped and draped in the usual sterile fashion with Betadine scrub and pain. Local infiltration with Polocaine 1% was used to achieve anesthesia. Using a #18-gauge needle, access was obtained into the right femoral vein. Over a guide wire, a 6-French sheath was advanced into this vessel. Using identical technique at 2 sites along the course of the right femoral vein, and through these sheaths, three 5-French, 5-mm quadripolar electrode catheters were advanced using fluoroscopic guidance. These 5-French, 5-mm quadripolar electrode catheters were advanced to positions in the high right atrium, right ventricular apex, and to a position across the tricuspid annulus such that a His bundle electrogram could be carefully mapped and recorded. After baseline intervals and pacing thresholds were obtained, RA and RV incremental pacing and programmed stimulation were performed. Sinus node recovery times were performed. Carotid sinus massage was performed. Gentle left-sided carotid sinus massage was associated with a systole of 6.5 seconds, a reproducible finding. At the end of the procedure, all catheters and sheaths were removed. He tolerated the procedure well.

s/b paint, typographical error

s/b asystole, Stedman's Medical Dictionary, 28E

FINDINGS:

1. At baseline, intracardiac intervals are normal with an AH interval of 50 msec and an HV interval of 54 msec.
2. Sinus node function is normal. All sinus node and all corrected sinus node recovery times are within normal limits. The longest corrected sinus node recovery time is normal at 166 msec.
3. AV nodal function is normal with an antegrade Wenckebach cycle length of 380 msec and an AV nodal refractory period of 550/300.

(continued)

4. No supraventricular arrhythmias were inducible.
5. Ventricular tachycardia is not inducible during this procedure, even with very aggressive pacing protocols. This includes RV incremental pacing and programmed stimulation at 2 sites, with 2 drive cycle lengths and up to 3 extra stimuli.
6. Marked carotid hypersensitivity is noted, with episodes of a systole of 6.5 seconds.

s/b are for uniformity in tense

s/b asystole, Stedman's Medical Dictionary, 28E

CONCLUSION:

This study is remarkable for marked carotid hypersensitivity with episodes of a systole associated with hypotension and a supine blood pressure of 75 mmHg.

RECOMMENDATIONS:

Given these findings, will recommend permanent pacemaker implantation.

For Signature

ABNORMAL ELECTROPHYSIOLOGIC STUDY

ELECTROPHYSIOLOGIC STUDY

PROCEDURE:

Electrophysiologic study.

CLINICAL HISTORY:

Syncope.

PROCEDURE/TECHNIQUE:

After informed consent was obtained, the patient was brought to the laboratory in a fasting state. He was prepped and draped in the usual sterile fashion with Betadine scrub and paint. Local infiltration with Polocaine 1% was used to achieve anesthesia. Using a #18-gauge needle, access was obtained into the right femoral vein. Over a guide wire, a 6-French sheath was advanced into this vessel. Using identical technique at 2 sites along the course of the right femoral vein, and through these sheaths, three 5-French, 5-mm quadripolar electrode catheters were advanced using fluoroscopic guidance. These 5-French, 5-mm quadripolar electrode catheters were advanced to positions in the high right atrium, right ventricular apex, and to a position across the tricuspid annulus such that a His bundle electrogram could be carefully mapped and recorded. After baseline intervals and pacing thresholds were obtained, RA and RV incremental pacing and programmed stimulation were performed. Sinus node recovery times were performed. Carotid sinus massage was performed. Gentle left-sided carotid sinus massage was associated with asystole of 6.5 seconds, a reproducible finding. At the end of the procedure, all catheters and sheaths were removed. He tolerated the procedure well.

FINDINGS:

1. At baseline, intracardiac intervals are normal with an AH interval of 50 msec and an HV interval of 54 msec.
2. Sinus node function is normal. All sinus node and all corrected sinus node recovery times are within normal limits. The longest corrected sinus node recovery time is normal at 166 msec.
3. AV nodal function is normal with an antegrade Wenckebach cycle length of 380 msec and an AV nodal refractory period of 550/300.
4. No supraventricular arrhythmias are inducible.
5. Ventricular tachycardia is not inducible during this procedure, even with very aggressive pacing protocols. This includes RV incremental pacing and programmed stimulation at 2 sites, with 2 drive cycle lengths and up to 3 extra stimuli.
6. Marked carotid hypersensitivity is noted, with episodes of asystole of 6.5 seconds.

CONCLUSION:

This study is remarkable for marked carotid hypersensitivity with episodes of asystole associated with hypotension and a supine blood pressure of 75 mmHg.

RECOMMENDATIONS:

Given these findings, will recommend permanent pacemaker implantation.

Answer Key

TRANSLUMINAL ANGIOPLASTY AND ANGIOGRAPHY

VASCULAR INTERVENTIONAL PROCEDURE

PROCEDURE:

1. Right axillary artery percutaneous transluminal angioplasty and angiogram.
2. Right common iliac artery percutaneous transluminal angioplasty and angiogram.
3. Unsuccessful right common femoral artery percutaneous transluminal angioplasty and angiogram.

CLINICAL HISTORY:

Patient is a 77-year-old female with bilateral leg claudication, right worse than the left.

TECHNIQUE:

Consent was obtained after explaining the risks, benefits, and alternatives, risks involving renal failure, retroperitoneal hemorrhage, bleeding, stroke, and imponderables. Single-stick access was gained in the right brachial artery. A 5-French sheath was placed. At this time, we tried to pass a wire into the subclavian artery, however, we could not make it pass into the artery at this time. Angiogram revealed a 70% focal short stenosis of the axillary artery. At this time, we placed a glide wire across the stenosis in the right axillary artery. This was followed by PTA with a 5 x 40 OPTA PRO balloon. It was inflated to 10 atmospheres for 90 seconds; stenosis was reduced from 70% to 20% with no evidence of dissection or embolization. Prior to this, Angiomax had been administered.

At this time, with the help of a LIMA catheter and a glide wire, we gained access into the distal abdominal aorta. We switched to a 0.035 non-glide J wire and placed a 90-mm Brite Tip sheath from the right side to the left distal abdominal aorta. With the help of a 5-French angled glide catheter and straight glide wire, and with great difficulty due to extreme tortuosity, we were able to gain access into the common femoral artery. Over a Quick Cross catheter, we placed a straight wire into the superficial femoral artery; however, at this time the Quick Cross catheter got stuck in the struts which were in the right femoral artery from before, which had a residual 40% to 50% stenosis. We had no luck in retrieving the catheter after multiple attempts.

(continued)

change comma to semicolon because *however* is used as a conjunctive adverb, AAMT Book of Style, however

s/b *Opta Pro*, use only initial capitals to avoid undue attention to the term, AAMT Book of Style, names, proprietary product names

Following that, we gained access into the right common iliac artery after dilating with a 5-French dilator. We were able to place a 7-French, 35-mm Brite Tip sheath into the common iliac artery. We placed a J wire into the distal abdominal aorta. This was followed by PTA of the common iliac artery with a 7 x 40 OPTA PRO balloon to 10 atmospheres for 60 seconds. The balloon was withdrawn. Angiogram revealed persistent 30% residual stenosis. At this time, we were able to successfully retrieve that Quick Cross catheter intact, with nothing embolized distally.

We decided to stop and recommend surgery for her right common femoral artery stenosis.

IMPRESSION:

1. Successful percutaneous transluminal angioplasty of the right axillary artery and right common femoral artery.
2. Unsuccessful percutaneous transluminal angioplasty of the right common femoral artery.

PLAN:

At this point, I would recommend patient undergo patch angioplasty of the right common femoral artery with a femorofemoral bypass surgery.

s/b Opta Pro, use only initial capitals to avoid undue attention to the term, AAMT Book of Style, names, proprietary product names

s/b iliac based on the text of the report

For Signature

TRANSLUMINAL ANGIOPLASTY AND ANGIOGRAPHY

VASCULAR INTERVENTIONAL PROCEDURE

PROCEDURE:

1. Right axillary artery percutaneous transluminal angioplasty and angiogram.
2. Right common iliac artery percutaneous transluminal angioplasty and angiogram.
3. Unsuccessful right common femoral artery percutaneous transluminal angioplasty and angiogram.

CLINICAL HISTORY:

Patient is a 77-year-old female with bilateral leg claudication, right worse than the left.

TECHNIQUE:

Consent was obtained after explaining the risks, benefits, and alternatives, risks involving renal failure, retroperitoneal hemorrhage, bleeding, stroke, and imponderables. Single-stick access was gained in the right brachial artery. A 5-French sheath was placed. At this time, we tried to pass a wire into the subclavian artery; however, we could not make it pass into the artery at this time. Angiogram revealed a 70% focal short stenosis of the axillary artery. At this time, we placed a glide wire across the stenosis in the right axillary artery. This was followed by PTA with a 5 x 40 Opta Pro balloon. It was inflated to 10 atmospheres for 90 seconds; stenosis was reduced from 70% to 20% with no evidence of dissection or embolization. Prior to this, Angiomax had been administered.

At this time, with the help of a LIMA catheter and a glide wire, we gained access into the distal abdominal aorta. We switched to a 0.035 non-glide J wire and placed a 90-mm Brite Tip sheath from the right side to the left distal abdominal aorta. With the help of a 5-French angled glide catheter and straight glide wire, and with great difficulty due to extreme tortuosity, we were able to gain access into the common femoral artery. Over a Quick Cross catheter, we placed a straight wire into the superficial femoral artery; however, at this time the Quick Cross catheter got stuck in the struts which were in the right femoral artery from before, which had a residual 40% to 50% stenosis. We had no luck in retrieving the catheter after multiple attempts.

Following that, we gained access into the right common iliac artery after dilating with a 5-French dilator. We were able to place a 7-French, 35-mm Brite Tip sheath into the common iliac artery. We placed a J wire into the distal abdominal aorta. This was followed by PTA of the common iliac artery with a 7 x 40 Opta Pro balloon to 10 atmospheres for 60 seconds. The balloon was withdrawn. Angiogram revealed persistent 30% residual stenosis. At this time, we were able to successfully retrieve that Quick Cross catheter intact, with nothing embolized distally.

We decided to stop and recommend surgery for her right common femoral artery stenosis.

(continued)

IMPRESSION:

1. Successful percutaneous transluminal angioplasty of the right axillary artery and right common iliac artery.
2. Unsuccessful percutaneous transluminal angioplasty of the right common femoral artery.

PLAN:

At this point, I would recommend patient undergo patch angioplasty of the right common femoral artery with a femorofemoral bypass surgery.

Answer Key   Report #43

CARDIAC CATHETERIZATION WITH VEIN GRAFT AND LEFT INTERNAL MAMMARY GRAFT ANGIOGRAPHY

OPERATIVE REPORT

TITLE OF PROCEDURE:
1. Left heart catheterization.
2. Coronary angiography.
3. Left ventriculography.
4. Saphenous vein graft angiography.
5. Left internal mammary graft angiography.

PROCEDURE IN DETAIL:
After informed consent was obtained and premedications administered, the area of the right femoral triangle was prepped and draped in the usual sterile fashion. Xylocaine 1% was used for local anesthesia. Modified seldinger technique was used to place a 6-French Hemaquet in the right femoral artery. Using standard Judkins technique with a JL4 and JR4, left followed by right coronary angiography was performed in multiple right anterior oblique and left anterior oblique views. The right coronary catheter was used for angiography of the internal mammary. A multipurpose catheter was used for right coronary artery saphenous vein graft angiography. Finally, a pigtail catheter was used for left ventriculography performed in the 30-degree RAO view. VasoSeal was used for hemostasis. The patient tolerated the procedure well. There were no complications.

s/b Seldinger, capitalize eponym, AAMT Book of Style, eponyms

The patient remained in a sinus rhythm. Left ventricular end-diastolic pressure was 16.

There was no gradient between the left ventricle and aorta on pullback. Left ventriculography revealed mild global hypokinesis but low normal left ventricular systolic function.

s/b low-normal, insert hyphen, AAMT Book of Style, compound modifiers

CORONARY ANGIOGRAPHY:
Injection of the left coronary system demonstrates a left main which trifurcates into an LAD, ramus and circumflex. Left main has a concentric 60% to 70% distal narrowing involving the trifurcation of the LAD, ramus and circumflex. There is no damping or ventricularization with catheter engagement.

The LAD is a fair-caliber vessel which gives rise to a moderate-size proximal diagonal and multiple septal perforating branches, and the LAD terminates just at the inferior aspect of the left ventricular

(continued)

apex. There is competitive spilling from the mid to distal LAD via the internal mammary bypass. The mid to distal LAD is widely patent and of fair-caliber. There is luminal irregularity in the proximal LAD with no obstructive lesions. Likewise, the first diagonal has diffuse irregularity but no obstructive disease.

The ramus is of smaller caliber and free of obstructive disease.

The right coronary artery is dominant and completely occluded near its origin.

SAPHENOUS VEIN GRAFT TO THE POSTERIOR DESCENDING ARTERY:
This graft is widely patent, briskly filling a fair-caliber PDA and a larger posterolateral system. There is some mild luminal irregularity, but no obstructive disease in this system.

s/b fair caliber, delete hyphen, AAMT Book of Style, hyphens, adjectives

For Signature

CARDIAC CATHETERIZATION WITH VEIN GRAFT AND LEFT INTERNAL MAMMARY GRAFT ANGIOGRAPHY

OPERATIVE REPORT

TITLE OF PROCEDURE:

6. Left heart catheterization.
7. Coronary angiography.
8. Left ventriculography.
9. Saphenous vein graft angiography.
10. Left internal mammary graft angiography.

PROCEDURE IN DETAIL:

After informed consent was obtained and premedications administered, the area of the right femoral triangle was prepped and draped in the usual sterile fashion. Xylocaine 1% was used for local anesthesia. Modified Seldinger technique was used to place a 6-French Hemaquet in the right femoral artery. Using standard Judkins technique with a JL4 and JR4, left followed by right coronary angiography was performed in multiple right anterior oblique and left anterior oblique views. The right coronary catheter was used for angiography of the internal mammary. A multipurpose catheter was used for right coronary artery saphenous vein graft angiography. Finally, a pigtail catheter was used for left ventriculography performed in the 30-degree RAO view. VasoSeal was used for hemostasis. The patient tolerated the procedure well. There were no complications.

The patient remained in a sinus rhythm. Left ventricular end-diastolic pressure was 16.

There was no gradient between the left ventricle and aorta on pullback. Left ventriculography revealed mild global hypokinesis but low-normal left ventricular systolic function.

CORONARY ANGIOGRAPHY:

Injection of the left coronary system demonstrates a left main which trifurcates into an LAD, ramus and circumflex. Left main has a concentric 60% to 70% distal narrowing involving the trifurcation of the LAD, ramus and circumflex. There is no damping or ventricularization with catheter engagement.

The LAD is a fair-caliber vessel which gives rise to a moderate-size proximal diagonal and multiple septal perforating branches, and the LAD terminates just at the inferior aspect of the left ventricular apex. There is competitive spilling from the mid to distal LAD via the internal mammary bypass. The mid to distal LAD is widely patent and of fair caliber. There is luminal irregularity in the proximal LAD with no obstructive lesions. Likewise, the first diagonal has diffuse irregularity but no obstructive disease.

The ramus is of smaller caliber and free of obstructive disease.

The right coronary artery is dominant and completely occluded near its origin.

SAPHENOUS VEIN GRAFT TO THE POSTERIOR DESCENDING ARTERY:

This graft is widely patent, briskly filling a fair-caliber PDA and a larger posterolateral system. There is some mild luminal irregularity but no obstructive disease in this system.

Answer Key

CORONARY ARTERY BYPASS GRAFT

OPERATIVE REPORT

TITLE OF PROCEDURE: Coronary artery bypass graft (CABG).

PROCEDURE IN DETAIL: The patient was brought to the operating room and given general endotracheal anesthesia. The pulmonary artery catheter was inserted by Anesthesia under sterile technique in the right internal jugular vein. The distal right saphenous vein was harvested from the medial malleolus to just above the knee using multiple small serial incisions with skin bridges. It was a good-quality vein. The leg was closed in layers with 2-0 and 3-0 Vicryl, with 3-0 Vicryl subcuticular suture in the skin.

A midline sternotomy was performed. The patient was heparinized. The ascending aorta was found to be extremely calcified after opening the pericardium. There was diffuse atherosclerosis with visible plaque emanating from the ascending aorta. The aortic arch was cannulated beyond the ascending aorta. The atrium was cannulated, and the patient was placed on bypass. A vent was inserted into the left ventricle via the right superior pulmonary vein. Coronaries were marked for bypass, including a very large posterior descending artery and a good-sized posterolateral branch just prior to its bifurcation with two smaller branches. A single-clamp technique was utilized. The aorta was crossclamped in the least calcified place. One liter of cardioplegia was given antegrade to arrest the heart. It was packed with ice and then flushed posteriorly.

Bypasses were accomplished, first using the reverse saphenous vein in an end-to-side fashion to the PDA, which was a good-quality 2.5 to 3-mm vessel. This was done with a reverse vein and running 7-0 Prolene suture. The second bypass was to the posterolateral branch, which was smaller but easily took a 1.5-mm probe. This was done with a separate piece of vein and a running 7-0 Prolene suture. A bolus of cold cardioplegia was given, and the patient was rewarmed. With the crossclamp still in place, a single aortotomy was made in the ascending aorta. The area was thickened and calcified but had a decent lumen to allow suture of the proximal end of the PDA up to the ascending aorta with running 5-0 Prolene suture in an end-to-side fashion. After concluding this anastomosis, hot cardioplegia was given into the aortic root. The crossclamp was removed after a total of 30 minutes crossclamp time. The remaining proximal anastomosis

(continued)

NOTE: capitalize a department name that is referred to as an entity, AAMT Book of Style, business names, departments

s/b 2.5-, insert hyphen, AAMT Book of Style, hyphens, suspensive

alt.: *cross-clamp*, Stedman's Cardiovascular and Pulmonary Words, 4E of the posterolateral branch was brought onto the hood of the PDA graft. The PDA was isolated with bulldog clamps. Venotomy was made, and the end-to-side anastomosis of the posterior left ventricle to the PDA was accomplished using running 6-0 Prolene suture in an end-to-side fashion. The system was back bled and de-aired, and the bulldog clamps were removed. Vessels were inspected, and they were both hemostatic.

s/b back-bled, insert hyphen, Stedman's Cardiovascular & Pulmonary Words, 4E, back-bleeding

s/b Two, AAMT Book of Style, numbers, beginning of a sentence

2 atrial and 2 ventricular pacing wires were placed and brought out through the skin. One single chest tube was placed into the mediastinum. Neither pleura was opened. The left ventricular vent was clamped and removed, and the pursestring was ligated. The lungs were inflated. The patient was ventilated and weaned off bypass successfully without the aid of inotropic support. Protamine was started and the atrial cannula was removed. Volume status was normalized and the heparin fully reversed with protamine. The aortic cannula was removed and the site ligated and reinforced with pledgeted 4-0 Prolene stitch. The chest tube was positioned. The wound was closed using figure-of-eight 0 Ethibond to reapproximate fascia, 7 sternal wires, and 2 layers of running 2-0 Vicryl and a running 3-0 Vicryl in the skin. The patient tolerated the procedure and was transferred to the intensive care unit in stable condition.

For Signature

CORONARY ARTERY BYPASS GRAFT

OPERATIVE REPORT

TITLE OF PROCEDURE: Coronary artery bypass graft (CABG).

PROCEDURE IN DETAIL: The patient was brought to the operating room and given general endotracheal anesthesia. The pulmonary artery catheter was inserted by Anesthesia under sterile technique in the right internal jugular vein. The distal right saphenous vein was harvested from the medial malleolus to just above the knee using multiple small serial incisions with skin bridges. It was a good-quality vein. The leg was closed in layers with 2-0 and 3-0 Vicryl, with 3-0 Vicryl subcuticular suture in the skin.

A midline sternotomy was performed. The patient was heparinized. The ascending aorta was found to be extremely calcified after opening the pericardium. There was diffuse atherosclerosis with visible plaque emanating from the ascending aorta. The aortic arch was cannulated beyond the ascending aorta. The atrium was cannulated, and the patient was placed on bypass. A vent was inserted into the left ventricle via the right superior pulmonary vein. Coronaries were marked for bypass, including a very large posterior descending artery and a good-sized posterolateral branch just prior to its bifurcation with two smaller branches. A single-clamp technique was utilized. The aorta was cross-clamped in the least calcified place. One liter of cardioplegia was given antegrade to arrest the heart. It was packed with ice and then flushed posteriorly.

Bypasses were accomplished, first using the reverse saphenous vein in an end-to-side fashion to the PDA, which was a good-quality 2.5- to 3-mm vessel. This was done with a reverse vein and running 7-0 Prolene suture. The second bypass was to the posterolateral branch, which was smaller but easily took a 1.5-mm probe. This was done with a separate piece of vein and a running 7-0 Prolene suture. A bolus of cold cardioplegia was given, and the patient was rewarmed. With the cross-clamp still in place, a single aortotomy was made in the ascending aorta. The area was thickened and calcified but had a decent lumen to allow suture of the proximal end of the PDA up to the ascending aorta with running 5-0 Prolene suture in an end-to-side fashion. After concluding this anastomosis, hot cardioplegia was given into the aortic root. The cross-clamp was removed after a total of 30 minutes cross-clamp time. The remaining proximal anastomosis of the posterolateral branch was brought onto the hood of the PDA graft. The PDA was isolated with bulldog clamps. Venotomy was made, and the end-to-side anastomosis of the posterior left ventricle to the PDA was accomplished using running 6-0 Prolene suture in an end-to-side fashion. The system was back-bled and de-aired, and the bulldog clamps were removed. Vessels were inspected, and they were both hemostatic.

Two atrial and 2 ventricular pacing wires were placed and brought out through the skin. One single chest tube was placed into the mediastinum. Neither pleura was opened. The left ventricular vent was clamped and removed, and the pursestring was ligated. The lungs were inflated. The patient was ventilated and weaned off bypass successfully without the aid of inotropic support. Protamine was started and the atrial cannula was removed. Volume status was normalized and the heparin

(continued)

fully reversed with protamine. The aortic cannula was removed and the site ligated and reinforced with pledgeted 4-0 Prolene stitch. The chest tube was positioned. The wound was closed using figure-of-eight 0 Ethibond to reapproximate fascia, 7 sternal wires, and 2 layers of running 2-0 Vicryl and a running 3-0 Vicryl in the skin. The patient tolerated the procedure and was transferred to the intensive care unit in stable condition.

Answer Key

DISCHARGE SUMMARY FOR ISCHEMIC CARDIOMYOPATHY

DISCHARGE SUMMARY

FINAL DIAGNOSES:
1. Ischemic cardiomyopathy
2. Status post defibrillator implantation
3. Ventricular tachycardia in 2004
4. History of amiodarone intolerance
5. Multiple defibrillator shocks
6. Hypertension
7. Hyperlipidemia
8. Status post initiation of mexiletine therapy for suppression of recurrent ventricular tachycardia that had resulted in shocks

insert periods after each diagnosis, AAMT Book of Style, lists, vertical lists

HOSPITAL COURSE: The patient was transferred from an outlying hospital due to multiple defibrillator shocks. He underwent loading on mexiletine after initially being placed on amiodarone. Amiodarone was discontinued due to a history of previous intolerance, including symptoms that were thought to be compatible with neuropathy. He tolerated loading with mexiletine well and was tested today, with excellent defibrillation thresholds.

s/b follow, typographical or dictation error

DISCHARGE INSTRUCTIONS: He will be discharged and will followed up with us in approximately 3 months.

s/b q. day, every day, or daily, ISMP List of Dangerous Abbreviations

DISCHARGE MEDICATIONS: Mexiletine 150 mg p.o. b.i.d. with meals, Plavix 75 mg p.o. q.d., aspirin 325 mg q.d., Vasotec 5 mg b.i.d., Toprol XL 50 mg b.i.d., Lanoxin 0.25 mg q.d., and folic acid 1 mg q.d.

s/b q. day, every day, or daily, ISMP List of Dangerous Abbreviations

For Signature

DISCHARGE SUMMARY FOR ISCHEMIC CARDIOMYOPATHY

DISCHARGE SUMMARY

FINAL DIAGNOSES:
1. Ischemic cardiomyopathy.
2. Status post defibrillator implantation.
3. Ventricular tachycardia in 2004.
4. History of amiodarone intolerance.
5. Multiple defibrillator shocks.
6. Hypertension.
7. Hyperlipidemia.
8. Status post initiation of mexiletine therapy for suppression of recurrent ventricular tachycardia that had resulted in shocks.

HOSPITAL COURSE: The patient was transferred from an outlying hospital due to multiple defibrillator shocks. He underwent loading on mexiletine after initially being placed on amiodarone. Amiodarone was discontinued due to a history of previous intolerance, including symptoms that were thought to be compatible with neuropathy. He tolerated loading with mexiletine well and was tested today, with excellent defibrillation thresholds.

DISCHARGE INSTRUCTIONS: He will be discharged and will follow up with us in approximately 3 months.

DISCHARGE MEDICATIONS: Mexiletine 150 mg p.o. b.i.d. with meals, Plavix 75 mg p.o. q. day, aspirin 325 mg q. day, Vasotec 5 mg b.i.d., Toprol-XL 50 mg b.i.d., Lanoxin 0.25 mg q. day, and folic acid 1 mg q. day.

Answer Key

AORTIC ARCH ANGIOGRAPHY

VASCULAR IMAGING STUDY

PROCEDURE: Aortic arch angiography, selective bilateral carotid angiography with cerebral angiography. Selective bilateral vertebral angiography with cerebral angiography. Angio-Seal deployment.

IDENTIFYING DATA: Patient is a 65-year-old Hispanic female with noninvasive evidence of high-grade stenosis at the origin of the right internal carotid artery.

DESCRIPTION: After informed consent was obtained, the patient was brought to the catheterization laboratory where the right groin was sterilely prepped and draped, and then anesthetized with Xylocaine. A 5-French sheath was placed in the RFA. An aortic arch angiogram was performed using a 5-French pigtail catheter. A 5-French angled glide catheter was then advanced to the right common carotid artery using an angled 0.035 glide wire. Selective carotid angiography was performed. Straight-lateral and AP-cranial cerebral angiograms were obtained during right carotid injection. The catheter was then redirected into the origin of the right vertebral artery, and right vertebral angiography was obtained. A posterior cerebral angiogram was obtained during right vertebral injection. Catheter was redirected into the left common carotid artery, and left carotid angiography was performed in multiple views. Straight-lateral and AP-cranial cerebral angiograms were obtained during left carotid injection. The catheter was then manipulated into the origin of the left vertebral artery. Left vertebral angiography was obtained. Posterior circulation cerebral angiography was obtained in the AP-cranial view. The catheter was removed. A 6-French Angio-Seal device was deployed, with satisfactory hemostasis.

COMPLICATIONS: None.

FLUOROSCOPY TIME: 5.3 minutes.

CONTRAST: 115 mL.

RESULTS:

1. Aortic arch angiography: The aortic arch is unremarkable. The common carotid arteries appear normal. The right innominate artery, right subclavian artery, as well as left

(continued)

subclavian artery, all appear normal. Vertebral arteries are patent bilaterally with the left vertebral artery appearing larger than the right.

2. Carotid angiography: The right internal carotid artery has a 95% osteal stenosis. The external carotid is normal. The left internal carotid artery has 40% to 50% osteal stenosis. There is 90% osteal stenosis of the left external carotid artery.

3. Vertebral angiography: The vertebral arteries are normal bilaterally.

4. Cerebral angiography: The anterior, middle, and posterior cerebral arteries all appear normal bilaterally. Posterior circulation is intact, with filling more from the left vertebral then from the right vertebral. No occlusive disease or aneurysm was identified.

FINAL IMPRESSION: Critical 95% stenosis at the origin of the right internal carotid artery. There is moderate 50% stenosis at the origin of the left internal carotid artery. Incidental note is made of left external carotid artery stenosis. Cerebral angiogram is unremarkable.

PLAN: Vascular surgical consultation, to access for revascularization.

s/b ostial, incorrect term, Stedman's Medical Dictionary, 28E

s/b ostial, incorrect term, Stedman's Medical Dictionary, 28E

s/b than, usage is comparative, general rule of grammar

s/b assess, incorrect term

For Signature

AORTIC ARCH ANGIOGRAPHY

VASCULAR IMAGING STUDY

PROCEDURE: Aortic arch angiography, selective bilateral carotid angiography with cerebral angiography. Selective bilateral vertebral angiography with cerebral angiography. Angio-Seal deployment.

IDENTIFYING DATA: Patient is a 65-year-old Hispanic female with noninvasive evidence of high-grade stenosis at the origin of the right internal carotid artery.

DESCRIPTION: After informed consent was obtained, the patient was brought to the catheterization laboratory where the right groin was sterilely prepped and draped, and then anesthetized with Xylocaine. A 5-French sheath was placed in the RFA. An aortic arch angiogram was performed using a 5-French pigtail catheter. A 5-French angled glide catheter was then advanced to the right common carotid artery using an angled 0.035 glide wire. Selective carotid angiography was performed. Straight-lateral and AP-cranial cerebral angiograms were obtained during right carotid injection. The catheter was then redirected into the origin of the right vertebral artery, and right vertebral angiography was obtained. A posterior cerebral angiogram was obtained during right vertebral injection. Catheter was redirected into the left common carotid artery, and left carotid angiography was performed in multiple views. Straight-lateral and AP-cranial cerebral angiograms were obtained during left carotid injection. The catheter was then manipulated into the origin of the left vertebral artery. Left vertebral angiography was obtained. Posterior circulation cerebral angiography was obtained in the AP-cranial view. The catheter was removed. A 6-French Angio-Seal device was deployed, with satisfactory hemostasis.

COMPLICATIONS: None.

FLUOROSCOPY TIME: 5.3 minutes.

CONTRAST: 115 mL.

RESULTS:
1. Aortic arch angiography: The aortic arch is unremarkable. The common carotid arteries appear normal. The right innominate artery, right subclavian artery, as well as left subclavian artery, all appear normal. Vertebral arteries are patent bilaterally with the left vertebral artery appearing larger than the right.
2. Carotid angiography: The right internal carotid artery has a 95% ostial stenosis. The external carotid is normal. The left internal carotid artery has 40% to 50% ostial stenosis. There is 90% ostial stenosis of the left external carotid artery.
3. Vertebral angiography: The vertebral arteries are normal bilaterally.
4. Cerebral angiography: The anterior, middle, and posterior cerebral arteries all appear normal bilaterally. Posterior circulation is intact, with filling more from the left vertebral than from the right vertebral. No occlusive disease or aneurysm was identified.

FINAL IMPRESSION: Critical 95% stenosis at the origin of the right internal carotid artery. There is moderate 50% stenosis at the origin of the left internal carotid artery. Incidental note is made of left external carotid artery stenosis. Cerebral angiogram is unremarkable.

PLAN: Vascular surgical consultation, to assess for revascularization.

Answer Key

RADIOFREQUENCY ABLATION

ELECTROPHYSIOLOGY INTERVENTION STUDY

PROCEDURE: Radiofrequency ablation.

CLINICAL HISTORY: A very pleasant 74-year-old woman with very rapid response to atrial fibrillation that has been refractory to aggressive attempts at antiarrhythmic management including Rythmol, Tambocor, amiodarone. She is aware of the risks, benefits and alternatives to proceeding with radiofrequency ablation and subsequent permanent pacemaker implantation during the electrophysiologic study. She understands and wishes to proceed.

TECHNIQUE: After informed consent was obtained, patient was brought to the electrophysiology laboratory in a fasting state. She was prepped and draped in the usual sterile fashion with multiple layers of Betadine. Lidocaine 1% infiltration was used to achieve local anesthesia in the right inguinal area. Using a #18-gauge needle, access was obtained into the left femoral vein. Over a guide wire, a 6-French sheath was advanced into this vessel. Using identical technique at a separate site along the course of the right femoral vein, a 7-French sheath was advanced. Through these sheaths, a 5-French 5-mm quadripolar electrode catheter was advanced to a position in the right ventricular apex, and a 7-French 2.5-mm Cordis Webster D-curve mapping/ablation catheter was advanced to a position across the tricuspid annulus such that a His bundle electrogram could be carefully mapped and recorded. After baseline intervals and pacing thresholds were obtained, excessive endocardial mapping was performed in the region of the His bundle. Radiofrequency energy was then applied at the site of His bundle activation. This was associated with purposeful induction of iatrogenic complete heart block, with a junctional escape rhythm at 40. The patient was observed for some time and then started on an isoproterenol infusion, after which the above process was repeated. No AV conduction was present. The patient continued to have a junctional escape rhythm at 40. Temporary pacing was accomplished to the right ventricular lead until a permanent pacemaker, which had previously been scheduled, could be implanted. He tolerated the procedure quite well.

CONCLUSION: Successful radiofrequency ablation.

Will proceed with previously scheduled permanent pacemaker.

NOTE: *guidewire* is also acceptable, Stedman's Medical Dictionary, 28E

s/b right based on the text of the report

s/b extensive, incorrect term

s/b She, common dictation error

For Signature

RADIOFREQUENCY ABLATION

ELECTROPHYSIOLOGY INTERVENTION STUDY

PROCEDURE: Radiofrequency ablation.

CLINICAL HISTORY: A very pleasant 74-year-old woman with very rapid response to atrial fibrillation that has been refractory to aggressive attempts at antiarrhythmic management including Rythmol, Tambocor, amiodarone. She is aware of the risks, benefits and alternatives to proceeding with radiofrequency ablation and subsequent permanent pacemaker implantation during the electrophysiologic study. She understands and wishes to proceed.

TECHNIQUE: After informed consent was obtained, patient was brought to the electrophysiology laboratory in a fasting state. She was prepped and draped in the usual sterile fashion with multiple layers of Betadine. Lidocaine 1% infiltration was used to achieve local anesthesia in the right inguinal area. Using a #18-gauge needle, access was obtained into the right femoral vein. Over a guidewire, a 6-French sheath was advanced into this vessel. Using identical technique at a separate site along the course of the right femoral vein, a 7-French sheath was advanced. Through these sheaths, a 5-French 5-mm quadripolar electrode catheter was advanced to a position in the right ventricular apex, and a 7-French 2.5-mm Cordis Webster D-curve mapping/ablation catheter was advanced to a position across the tricuspid annulus such that a His bundle electrogram could be carefully mapped and recorded. After baseline intervals and pacing thresholds were obtained, extensive endocardial mapping was performed in the region of the His bundle. Radiofrequency energy was then applied at the site of His bundle activation. This was associated with purposeful induction of iatrogenic complete heart block, with a junctional escape rhythm at 40. The patient was observed for some time and then started on an isoproterenol infusion, after which the above process was repeated. No AV conduction was present. The patient continued to have a junctional escape rhythm at 40. Temporary pacing was accomplished to the right ventricular lead until a permanent pacemaker, which had previously been scheduled, could be implanted. She tolerated the procedure quite well.

CONCLUSION:

Successful radiofrequency ablation.

Will proceed with previously scheduled permanent pacemaker.

Answer Key

CARDIAC CATHETERIZATION WITH PUMP INSERTION AND PACEMAKER WIRE INSERTION

PACEMAKER REPORT

FINAL DIAGNOSES:
1. severe 3-vessel coronary artery disease
2. acute anterior subendocardial myocardial infarction
3. mild to moderate left ventricular systolic dysfunction

PROCEDURES PERFORMED:
1. cardiac catheterization
2. selective coronary arteriography
3. left ventriculography
4. intraaortic balloon pump insertion
5. temporary transvenous pacemaker wire insertion

INDICATIONS: This patient has acute subendocardial myocardial infarction.

DESCRIPTION OF PROCEDURE: The patient was prepped and draped in the usual sterile fashion. Versed 1 mg IV conscious sedation was given. Local anesthesia was then applied to the right groin. An 8-French sheath was placed in the right femoral artery without difficulty. A 6-French sheath was then placed in the right femoral vein without difficulty. The 6-French JL4 and 6-French JR4 diagnostic catheters were used to perform selective coronary arteriography in various LAO and RAO projections. Left ventriculogram in the RAO projection was then performed by advancing a pigtail catheter into the left ventricle. Continuous pressure monitoring was performed during pullback of this catheter across the aortic valve. Upon identification of the anatomy, an intraaortic balloon pump was inserted, and a temporary transvenous pacemaker wire was inserted.

LEFT MAIN: The left main coronary artery is a large-caliper vessel with minimal irregularities.

LEFT ANTERIOR DESCENDING: The LAD is a large-caliber vessel that gives rise to a moderate-sized first diagonal branch and small second diagonal branch. Following the origin of the first diagonal branch, there is a long 90% to 95% stenosis. There are filling defects within this lesion consistent with thrombus. The remainder of the mid LAD and distal LAD has some mild diffuse disease. The first diagonal branch has a proximal 40% stenosis and mild,

(continued)

Margin notes:

capitalize first letter of each entry, AAMT Book of Style, lists, vertical lists

insert period after each entry, AAMT Book of Style, lists, vertical lists

alt: insert heading *FINDINGS*:, AAMT Book of Style, formats; NOTE: always follow the format required by your facility

s/b *large-caliber*, incorrect term

diffuse disease. The second diagonal branch is a small vessel with a proximal 70% stenosis.

LEFT CIRCUMFLEX: The left circumflex coronary artery is a large, nondominant vessel. It is ectatic in appearance and gives rise to a moderate-sized first marginal branch and moderate-sized second bifurcating marginal branch. The second marginal branch has a 60% stenosis in both limbs of the bifurcation and mild, diffuse disease. The reminder of the circumflex has mild to moderate diffuse disease.

RIGHT CORONARY ARTERY: The RCA is a large, dominant vessel. It gives rise to a moderate-sized posterolateral branch and a moderate-sized posterior descending branch. In the mid right coronary artery there is a 40% eccentric stenosis. The ostium of the posterior descending artery is then narrowed by approximately 90%. The remainder of the PDA has only minimal irregularities.

LEFT VENTRICULOGRAM: Left ventricular systolic function is mildly to moderately diminished. Estimated ejection fraction is 40%. There is anterolateral severe hypokinesis. There is no mitral regurgitation. There is no gradient across the aortic valve. Left ventricular end-diastolic pressure is 22.

DEVICE INSERTION: Upon identification of the anatomy, the 8-French right femoral arterial sheath was exchanged for an 8-French balloon pump sheath. A 40-mL intraaortic balloon pump was then inserted in the usual fashion. A 5-French pacemaker wire was advanced through the right femoral venous sheath to the right ventricular apex and was tested. Testing of thresholds revealed threshold to be less than 0.5 mA. The pacemaker was then set for a backup rate of 40.

COMMENTS: Based on the patient's anatomy, a decision is made for the patient to undergo surgical revascularization. The cardiothoracic surgeon came to the catheterization laboratory and reviewed the images. He agreed this was a suitable strategy for the patient. Because the patient had received Plavix and Integrilin, it was felt that surgery should be delayed a period of hours to days to reduce bleeding risk. For that reason, an intraaortic balloon pump was inserted. Given what we believe is a new left anterior fascicular block and right bundle branch block, a temporary transvenous pacemaker wire was inserted.

For Signature

CARDIAC CATHETERIZATION WITH PUMP INSERTION AND PACEMAKER WIRE INSERTION

PACEMAKER REPORT

FINAL DIAGNOSES:
1. Severe 3-vessel coronary artery disease.
2. Acute anterior subendocardial myocardial infarction.
3. Mild to moderate left ventricular systolic dysfunction.

PROCEDURES PERFORMED:
1. Cardiac catheterization.
2. Selective coronary arteriography.
3. Left ventriculography.
4. Intraaortic balloon pump insertion.
5. Temporary transvenous pacemaker wire insertion.

INDICATIONS: This patient has acute subendocardial myocardial infarction.

DESCRIPTION OF PROCEDURE: The patient was prepped and draped in the usual sterile fashion. Versed 1 mg IV conscious sedation was given. Local anesthesia was then applied to the right groin. An 8-French sheath was placed in the right femoral artery without difficulty. A 6-French sheath was then placed in the right femoral vein without difficulty. The 6-French JL4 and 6-French JR4 diagnostic catheters were used to perform selective coronary arteriography in various LAO and RAO projections. Left ventriculogram in the RAO projection was then performed by advancing a pigtail catheter into the left ventricle. Continuous pressure monitoring was performed during pullback of this catheter across the aortic valve. Upon identification of the anatomy, an intraaortic balloon pump was inserted, and a temporary transvenous pacemaker wire was inserted.

FINDINGS:
LEFT MAIN: The left main coronary artery is a large-caliber vessel with minimal irregularities.

LEFT ANTERIOR DESCENDING: The LAD is a large-caliber vessel that gives rise to a moderate-sized first diagonal branch and small second diagonal branch. Following the origin of the first diagonal branch, there is a long 90% to 95% stenosis. There are filling defects within this lesion consistent with thrombus. The remainder of the mid LAD and distal LAD has some mild diffuse disease. The first diagonal branch has a proximal 40% stenosis and mild, diffuse disease. The second diagonal branch is a small vessel with a proximal 70% stenosis.

LEFT CIRCUMFLEX: The left circumflex coronary artery is a large, nondominant vessel. It is ectatic in appearance and gives rise to a moderate-sized first marginal branch and moderate-sized second bifurcating marginal branch. The second marginal branch has a 60% stenosis in both limbs of the bifurcation and mild, diffuse disease. The reminder of the circumflex has mild to moderate diffuse disease.

(continued)

RIGHT CORONARY ARTERY: The RCA is a large, dominant vessel. It gives rise to a moderate-sized posterolateral branch and a moderate-sized posterior descending branch. In the mid right coronary artery there is a 40% eccentric stenosis. The ostium of the posterior descending artery is then narrowed by approximately 90%. The remainder of the PDA has only minimal irregularities.

LEFT VENTRICULOGRAM: Left ventricular systolic function is mildly to moderately diminished. Estimated ejection fraction is 40%. There is anterolateral severe hypokinesis. There is no mitral regurgitation. There is no gradient across the aortic valve. Left ventricular end-diastolic pressure is 22.

DEVICE INSERTION: Upon identification of the anatomy, the 8-French right femoral arterial sheath was exchanged for an 8-French balloon pump sheath. A 40-mL intraaortic balloon pump was then inserted in the usual fashion. A 5-French pacemaker wire was advanced through the right femoral venous sheath to the right ventricular apex and was tested. Testing of thresholds revealed threshold to be less than 0.5 mA. The pacemaker was then set for a backup rate of 40.

COMMENTS: Based on the patient's anatomy, a decision is made for the patient to undergo surgical revascularization. The cardiothoracic surgeon came to the catheterization laboratory and reviewed the images. He agreed this was a suitable strategy for the patient. Because the patient had received Plavix and Integrilin, it was felt that surgery should be delayed a period of hours to days to reduce bleeding risk. For that reason, an intraaortic balloon pump was inserted. Given what we believe is a new left anterior fascicular block and right bundle branch block, a temporary transvenous pacemaker wire was inserted.

Answer Key

INSERTION OF TRANSVENOUS TEMPORARY PACEMAKER

PACEMAKER REPORT

TITLE OF PROCEDURE: Insertion of transvenous temporary pacemaker by right internal jugular route.

PROCEDURE IN DETAIL: A right jugular stick following Xylocaine anesthesia was made in the triangle between the medial and lateral heads of the trapezius muscles. The internal jugular vein was cannulated initially with needles, using a guidewire. An Arrow introducer sheath was placed. The transvenous pacemaker selected was 3-French. The introducer sheath required a 5-French catheter to maintain a good seal. Intravenous fluid was infused via the side ports of the catheter following good venous return.

The transvenous balloon-type catheter, a flow-directed catheter but without capability of hemodynamic monitoring, was inserted with balloon up to approximately 45 cm and then manipulated between 52 cm from the introducer up to 32 cm from the introducer with best capture seen at 32 cm. Partial capturing was seen at settings at 0.5 mA to 1 mA with good capture at 2 mA. The rate was set at 60 beats per minute with complete capturing. Steri-Strips were used to wrap around the external portion of the catheter, and the catheter was secured to the introducer site port tubing. X-ray was taken showing the tip of the catheter within the right ventricle in good position.

---

s/b 3 French, delete hyphen, only hyphenate if the compound precedes the noun it modifies, AAMT Book of Style, compound modifiers, numerals with words

---

NOTE: *beats per minute* is commonly abbreviated to *BPM* or *bpm*, AAMT Book of Style, beats per minute

For Signature

INSERTION OF TRANSVENOUS TEMPORARY PACEMAKER

PACEMAKER REPORT

TITLE OF PROCEDURE: Insertion of transvenous temporary pacemaker by right internal jugular route.

PROCEDURE IN DETAIL: A right jugular stick following Xylocaine anesthesia was made in the triangle between the medial and lateral heads of the trapezius muscles. The internal jugular vein was cannulated initially with needles, using a guidewire. An Arrow introducer sheath was placed. The transvenous pacemaker selected was 3 French. The introducer sheath required a 5-French catheter to maintain a good seal. Intravenous fluid was infused via the side ports of the catheter following good venous return.

The transvenous balloon-type catheter, a flow-directed catheter but without capability of hemodynamic monitoring, was inserted with balloon up to approximately 45 cm and then manipulated between 52 cm from the introducer up to 32 cm from the introducer with best capture seen at 32 cm. Partial capturing was seen at settings at 0.5 mA to 1 mA with good capture at 2 mA. The rate was set at 60 bpm with complete capturing. Steri-Strips were used to wrap around the external portion of the catheter, and the catheter was secured to the introducer site port tubing. X-ray was taken showing the tip of the catheter within the right ventricle in good position.

Answer Key

Report #50

IMPLANTATION OF CARDIOVERTER DEFIBRILLATOR

NOTE: Ragged-right margins are preferred over right-justified margins, with all lines flush left (block format), AAMT Book of Style, formats

CARDIOLOGY PROCEDURE REPORT

PROCEDURES:
1. Implantation of an implantable cardioverter defibrillator.
2. Defibrillation threshold testing.
3. Final programming of the device.

PREPROCEDURE DIAGNOSIS: Ventricular tachycardia.

POSTPROCEDURE DIAGNOSIS: Ventricular tachycardia.

ANESTHESIA: Diprivan.

COMPLICATIONS: None.

DEFIBRILLATOR GENERATOR: Guidant Ventak Mini IV model #1790, serial #XXXXXX.

DEFIBRILLATOR LEAD: Intermedics model #497-23-70, serial #XXXXX, single-coil defibrillator lead.

BRIEF HISTORY: The patient is a 64-year-old white male who has a history of ischemic cardiomyopathy. he had ventricular tachycardia preoperatively and was found to have triple-vessel coronary disease. He underwent 6-vessel bypass surgery and underwent postoperative electrophysiologic study which revealed reliably induced ventricular fibrillation with his developing sustained monomorphic ventricular tachycardia after infusion of intravenous procainamide. Because of this, it was recommended that a defibrillator be placed.

s/b He, capitalize the first word of a sentence, general rule of grammer

PROCEDURE: After informed consent was signed, the patient was brought to the electrophysiology laboratory, and the left infraclavicular area was prepped and draped in the usual sterile fashion. The area was infused with 1% Xylocaine, and a defibrillator pocket was formed with the incision made parallel from the left clavicle down to the level of the prepectoral fascia. The left subclavian vein was then easily cannulated, and over a guidewire a 10.5-French sheath was passed without difficulty. Through this sheath an Intermedics model #497-23-70 single coil tined defibrillator lead was passed under fluoroscopic guidance to the left ventricular apex.

s/b single-coil, insert hyphen, AAMT Book of Style, hyphens, adjectives

(continued)

After adequate endocardial anchoring, threshold testing via the pacing system analyzer ensued: R waves measured 5.6 mV, ventricular capture down to an amplitude of 0.5 V, and a pulse width of 0.5 msec, measuring a current of 1.2 mA. The final volt resistance measured 400 ohms. Since these were felt to be appropriate pacing-sensing thresholds, the lead was anchored using the anchoring sleeve with two 2-0 Ethibond sutures. After this, the lead was attached to a CPI/Guidant Ventak Mini IV, model #1790, serial #XXXXXX, defibrillator. The defibrillator was set to detect ventricular fibrillation for any heart rate exceeding 180 beats per minute. Once attached, R waves measured 6.3 mV, impedance measured 416 ohms, and capture was less than 0.6 V, indicating appropriate connections.

The defibrillator and additional lead were then placed in the free-form pocket, and defibrillation threshold testing ensued:

Test #1: Using shock on T-wave algorithm, ventricular fibrillation was induced, and after 9.3 seconds a 17-joule shock was delivered which converted the arrhythmia to normal sinus rhythm. The shock impedance measured 88 ohms.

Test #2: Using similar simulation, ventricular fibrillation was induced, and after 8.8 seconds another 17-joule shock was delivered which promptly converted ventricular fibrillation to normal sinus rhythm. The shock impedance measured 82 ohms. These were felt to be appropriate responses with adequate impedances.

The defibrillator was left in position. The pocket was closed with two layers of 3-0 Vicryl sutures to the subcutaneous tissues and a single layer of 4-0 Vicryl sutures using a subcuticular stitch. Steri-Strips and a pressure dressing were then applied.

The patient was awaken from anesthesia and tolerated the procedure well. She was transferred to the progressive care unit in stable condition.

s/b He, based on the text of the report, common transcription error

s/b awakened, subject-verb agreement

CONCLUSIONS:
1. Successful implantation of a CPI Mini IV transvenous defibrillator and Intermedics single-coil ventricular lead.
2. Defibrillation threshold less than or equal to 17 joules.
3. Reliably induced ventricular fibrillation.
4. Final programming as mentioned above with the first shock energy set at 27 joules.

For Signature

IMPLANTATION OF CARDIOVERTER DEFIBRILLATOR

CARDIOLOGY PROCEDURE REPORT

PROCEDURES:
1. Implantation of an implantable cardioverter defibrillator.
2. Defibrillation threshold testing.
3. Final programming of the device.

PREPROCEDURE DIAGNOSIS: Ventricular tachycardia.

POSTPROCEDURE DIAGNOSIS: Ventricular tachycardia.

ANESTHESIA: Diprivan.

COMPLICATIONS: None.

DEFIBRILLATOR GENERATOR: Guidant Ventak Mini IV model #1790, serial #XXXXXX.

DEFIBRILLATOR LEAD: Intermedics model #497-23-70, serial #XXXXX, single-coil defibrillator lead.

BRIEF HISTORY: The patient is a 64-year-old white male who has a history of ischemic cardiomyopathy. He had ventricular tachycardia preoperatively and was found to have triple-vessel coronary disease. He underwent 6-vessel bypass surgery and underwent postoperative electrophysiologic study which revealed reliably induced ventricular fibrillation with his developing sustained monomorphic ventricular tachycardia after infusion of intravenous procainamide. Because of this, it was recommended that a defibrillator be placed.

PROCEDURE: After informed consent was signed, the patient was brought to the electrophysiology laboratory, and the left infraclavicular area was prepped and draped in the usual sterile fashion. The area was infused with 1% Xylocaine, and a defibrillator pocket was formed with the incision made parallel from the left clavicle down to the level of the prepectoral fascia. The left subclavian vein was then easily cannulated, and over a guidewire a 10.5-French sheath was passed without difficulty. Through this sheath an Intermedics model #497-23-70 single-coil tined defibrillator lead was passed under fluoroscopic guidance to the left ventricular apex.

After adequate endocardial anchoring, threshold testing via the pacing system analyzer ensued: R waves measured 5.6 mV, ventricular capture down to an amplitude of 0.5 V, and a pulse width of 0.5 msec, measuring a current of 1.2 mA. The final volt resistance measured 400 ohms. Since these were felt to be appropriate pacing-sensing thresholds, the lead was anchored using the anchoring sleeve with two 2-0 Ethibond sutures. After this, the lead was attached to a CPI/Guidant Ventak Mini IV, model #1790, serial #XXXXXX, defibrillator. The defibrillator was set to detect ventricular fibrillation for any heart rate exceeding 180 beats per minute. Once attached, R waves measured 6.3 mV, impedance measured 416 ohms, and capture was less than 0.6 V, indicating appropriate connections.

(continued)

The defibrillator and additional lead were then placed in the free-form pocket, and defibrillation threshold testing ensued:

Test #1: Using shock on T-wave algorithm, ventricular fibrillation was induced, and after 9.3 seconds a 17-joule shock was delivered which converted the arrhythmia to normal sinus rhythm. The shock impedance measured 88 ohms.

Test #2: Using similar simulation, ventricular fibrillation was induced, and after 8.8 seconds another 17-joule shock was delivered which promptly converted ventricular fibrillation to normal sinus rhythm. The shock impedance measured 82 ohms. These were felt to be appropriate responses with adequate impedances.

The defibrillator was left in position. The pocket was closed with two layers of 3-0 Vicryl sutures to the subcutaneous tissues and a single layer of 4-0 Vicryl sutures using a subcuticular stitch. Steri-Strips and a pressure dressing were then applied.

The patient was awakened from anesthesia and tolerated the procedure well. He was transferred to the progressive care unit in stable condition.

CONCLUSIONS:

1. Successful implantation of a CPI Mini IV transvenous defibrillator and Intermedics single-coil ventricular lead.
2. Defibrillation threshold less than or equal to 17 joules.
3. Reliably induced ventricular fibrillation.
4. Final programming as mentioned above with the first shock energy set at 27 joules.

Standard Proofreader's Marks

Mark	Action	Example	Result
ℐ	delete	remove this word	remove this
⊂	close up	clos e it up	close it up
ℐ	delete and close up	cl ose it up	close it up
⟨#⟩	add space; insert a space	give me somespace ⟨#⟩	give me some space
∧	caret; insert addition	add this here — word	add this word here
⟨stet⟩	leave as is	no changes to this are necessary ⟨stet⟩	no changes to this are necessary
¶	begin a new paragraph	This is the last sentence for this ¶ paragraph. This is the first sentence of the next paragraph.	This is the last sentence for this paragraph. This is the first sentence of the next paragraph.
⊙	insert a period	The sentence ends here ⊙	The sentence ends here.
∧	insert a comma	For this one add a comma	For this one, add a comma
∧	insert a semicolon	This is this however, that is that	This is this; however, that is that
∧	insert a colon	This list includes the following comma, semicolon, and colon	This list includes the following: comma, semicolon, and colon
=	insert a hyphen	one time thing	one-time thing
⟨lc⟩	change to lowercase	this WORD should not be capitalized ⟨lc⟩	this word should not be capitalized
⟨c+lc⟩	lowercase with initial capitals	this title should be capitalized ⟨c + lc⟩	This Title Should Be Capitalized
⟨caps⟩	set in large capitals	this word should be in all caps ⟨caps⟩	this WORD should be in all caps
[	move to left	[flush to the left	flush to the left
]	move to right	this line should be indented]	this line should be indented

Mark	Action	Example	Result
(tr)	transpose	change order the ⌐ (tr)	change the order
(?)	query to the author	this is confusing (?)	this is confusing
/	used to separate two or more marks and often used as a concluding stroke at the end of an insertion	insert period and delete this capitalize (c+lc) the first letter of the next sentence	insert period. Capitalize the first letter of the next sentence.
⌐	line break	break line here not elsewhere	break line here not elsewhere

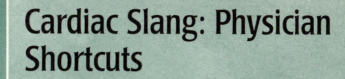

Cardiac Slang: Physician Shortcuts

Most physicians would rather be doing anything but dictating; hence, they devise unique ways to vocalize information, fully expecting the medical transcriptionist to know what they mean. Cardiologists frequently offer colorful word choices, especially while doing imaging and interventional procedures. It is not uncommon to hear that a catheter, wire, sheath, balloon, guide or stent has been parked, thrust, dithered, deployed, floated, pushed, inserted, finagled, teased, passed, re-passed, exchanged, crossed, coiled, curled, inflated, deflated, retrieved, tested, de-placed, replaced, tugged or kissed!

As per *The AAMT Book of Style for Medical Transcription, 2nd Edition*, slang terms and phrases used in dictation should be modified to reflect the medically correct term or phrase. This appendix will help you to navigate through some of the jargon and understand what is meant by the bizarre (*ax-fem-fem*), the frightening (*patient crashed*) and even the occasional farm animal reference (*went with a pig*).

Slang Term	Meaning
2 A's	two atrial pacing wires
accels	accelerations; pronounced *a-sells*
A-fib	atrial fibrillation
A-flutter	atrial flutter
angio	angiogram, angiography
angioplastiable	amenable to angioplasty, able to be angioplastied
antegradely	in antegrade fashion, antegrade flow
ax-fem-fem	axillofemoral-femoral (bypass)
bi-V	biventricular
bolused	gave/administered a bolus
brady down, brady'd down	experienced bradycardia
cath, cath'd	catheterization, catheterized
circ	circumflex
coags	coagulation studies
collateralized, collateralization	flowed from the collateral vessels, collateral flow

Slang Term	Meaning
crashed	arrested, coded
cues	Q waves
culotted	used the culotte technique
decels	decelerations; pronounced *de-sells*
defib	defibrillator, defibrillated
de-satting	desaturating
diag	diagonal
electro response	electrocardiographic response
eppy	epinephrine
fem-pop	femoropopliteal
hemo response	hemodynamic response
heparinized, heparinization	administered heparin, heparin administration
kegs	kilograms (kg)
kilo/kilos	kilogram/s (kg)
K-mag	potassium and magnesium
med telly	medical telemetry
migs	milligrams (mg)
mikes	micrograms (mcg)
nitro	nitroglycerin
nitroglycerins	nitroglycerin tablets
ox sat	oxygen saturation
pacer	pacemaker
pacer rep	pacemaker (manufacturer) representative
palp/palps	palpation/s
perf	perforation
pericardial stays	pericardial stay sutures
pig	pigtail catheter
P-thal	Persantine thallium (usually said as a study title)
pulse ox	pulse oximetry/oximeter
Q's	Q waves
retrogradely	in retrograde fashion, retrograde flow
rhoncherous sounds	rhonchi

Slang Term	Meaning
sats, satting	saturations, saturating
septal perf	septal perforator
swan	Swan-Ganz catheter
tacky	tachycardia, tachycardic
triple A	AAA (abbreviation for abdominal aortic aneurysm)
2 V's	two ventricular pacing wires
Valsalva'd	used the Valsalva maneuver
V-fib	ventricular fibrillation
V-gram	ventriculogram
V-tack	ventricular tachycardia

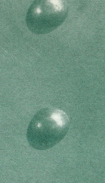

Cardiology Web Sites

Cardiology Information Resources

Web Site Address	Name	Description
http://www.acc.org	American College of Cardiology	Offers recent news, articles and research related to the field of cardiology. Includes links to educational programs, career sessions and job openings. Includes a link to sign up for an ACC membership as well as information on advocacy issues and summits offered by the organization.
http://www.angioplasty.org or http://www.ptca.org	Angioplasty.org	Provides information on interventional cardiology for both patients and professionals.
http://www.ecglibrary.com	ECG Library	Contains a collection of realistic looking electrocardiogram recordings.
http://www.mic.ki.se/diseases/C14.html	Karolinska Institute	Lists diseases and disorders pertaining to cardiovascular disease.
http://www.musc.edu	Medical University of South Carolina	Includes medical procedures, indications and descriptions of cardiac intervention. Also contains a glossary of terms and acronym expansions for perfusion technology, open heart surgery and cardiology.
http://www.musc.edu/perfusion/interven.htm	Medical University of South Carolina Cardiovascular Perfusion	Provides information on medical and surgical intervention for congenital and acquired cardiovascular disease.
http://www.nlm.nih.gov/medlineplus/druginformation.html	Medline Plus	Includes information on drugs, supplements and herbs.
http://www.medtronic.com/physician/cardiology.html	Medtronic	Contains a list of cardiac conditions, therapies and products.

Web Site Address	Name	Description
http://www.nhlbi.nih.gov/labs/7east/cardmeds.htm	National Heart, Lung, and Blood Institute	Lists cardiac medications by class.
http://www.sjm.com	St. Jude Medical	Includes information on conditions, procedures, devices and more.
http://www.theheart.org	The Heart.org	Offers articles regarding new technology and breakthroughs in cardiology. Free registration is available for those who would like to listen to the live presentations.
http://sln2.fi.edu/biosci/heart.html	The Franklin Institute Online	Details anatomy of the heart.
http://www.health.ucsd.edu/labref	University of California, San Diego, Medical Center	Contains laboratory values and procedures.
http://www.en.wikipedia.org/wiki/Defibrillator	Wikipedia	Showcases different types of defibrillators including internal and external defibrillators.

Manufacturers of Cardiology Equipment

Web Site Address	Name	Description
http://www.btlnet.com	BTL Industries Limited	Manufacture digital electrocardiographs, PC software for electrocardiographic monitoring, ergometry systems, electrocardiographic Holter monitors, and an ambulatory blood pressure Holter monitor for clinical practice.
http://www.cardiacscience.com	Cardiac Science Corp.	Develop, manufacture and market diagnostic and therapeutic cardiology products and services.
http://www.cardiodynamics.com	CardioDynamics International Corp.	Manufacture noninvasive hemodynamic monitoring and management systems.
http://www.datascope.com	DataScope Corp.	Manufacture proprietary products for clinical healthcare markets in anesthesiology, interventional cardiology, cardiovascular surgery and critical care medicine. Products include physiological monitors and cardiac assist systems.

Web Site Address	Name	Description
http://www.guidant.com/products	Guidant Corp.	Manufacture stents, defibrillators and other equipment and accessories used to treat coronary artery disease, bradyarrhythmias, tachyarrhythmias, atrial fibrillation, heart failure and more.
http://www.infimed.com	InfiMed Inc.	Manufacture a radiology and cardiology digital imaging system, angiographic digital imaging systems and a picture archival communications system.
http://www.medtronic.com/physician/cardsurgery.html	Medtronic Inc.	Manufacture equipment designed for arrested heart surgery, improved extracorporeal circulation and more.

Report Index

Note: Page numbers for reports in the Proofreading and Editing Exercises refer to the location of the final corrected (or "For Signature") report.

Report Topic	Section	Report #	Location
Angioplasty and Angiography (Transluminal)	Proofreading & Editing Exercises	42	page 271
Angioplasty (Balloon) of the Circumflex Coronary Artery, Coronary Angiography and	MT Practice	A-24	CD-ROM
Angioplasty (Balloon), Peripheral Atherectomy with	MT Practice	A-28	CD-ROM
Angioplasty (Kissing-Balloon Bilateral) of the Common Iliac Artery, Aortogram With Runoff and	MT Practice	A-22	CD-ROM
Angioplasty of the Subclavian Artery with Stenting	MT Practice	A-32	CD-ROM
Angioplasty (Percutaneous Transluminal) of the Left Femoral Artery, Abdominal Aortogram with Runoff and	MT Practice	A-26	CD-ROM
Annuloplasty (Complex Valve), Coronary Artery Bypass Graft, Radiofrequency Ablation, Transesophageal Echocardiography and Endoscopic Vein Harvest	MT Practice	A-43	CD-ROM
Aortic Arch Angiography	Proofreading & Editing Exercises	46	page 284
Aortic Arch Angiography, Carotid Angiography and Vertebral Angiography	MT Practice	A-17	CD-ROM
Aortic Cannulation, Stent Graft Repair and	MT Practice	A-44	CD-ROM
Aortogram (Abdominal) with Lower Extremity Runoff	Proofreading & Editing Exercises	5	page 159
Aortogram (Abdominal) with Runoff and Percutaneous Transluminal Angioplasty of the Left Femoral Artery	MT Practice	A-26	CD-ROM
Aortogram with Runoff and Kissing-Balloon Bilateral Common Iliac Artery Angioplasty	MT Practice	A-22	CD-ROM
Arteriography (Thoracic Arch) to Visualize Carotid Arteries	Proofreading & Editing Exercises	8	page 166
Atherectomy (Peripheral) with Balloon Angioplasty	MT Practice	A-28	CD-ROM
Atrial Fibrillation, History and Physical Examination for	Proofreading & Editing Exercises	11	page 176
Atrioventricular Canal Repair with Ligation of Patent Ductus Arteriosus	Proofreading & Editing Exercises	27	page 227

Report Topic	Section	Report #	Location
Band Adjustment and Shunt Ligation (Pediatric)	MT Practice	A-50	CD-ROM
Bilateral Lower Extremity Venous Doppler Study of Patient with Deep Venous Thrombosis	MT Practice	A-5	CD-ROM
Biventricular Implantable Cardioverter-Defibrillator Placement	MT Practice	A-49	CD-ROM
Bypass, Consultation for Evaluation of Suitability for	Proofreading & Editing Exercises	15	page 190
Cardiac Catheterization with Pump Insertion and Pacemaker Wire Insertion	Proofreading & Editing Exercises	48	page 289
Cardiac Catheterization with Vein Graft and Left Internal Mammary Graft Angiography	Proofreading & Editing Exercises	43	page 275
Cardiac Duplex Imaging Study	MT Practice	A-10	CD-ROM
Cardiomyopathy, Left Heart Catheterization and Ventriculography in Patient with	Proofreading & Editing Exercises	21	page 209
Cardiothoracic Surgical Consultation for Evaluation of Suitability for Bypass	Proofreading & Editing Exercises	15	page 190
Cardioversion (Electrical)	Proofreading & Editing Exercises	38	page 261
Cardioversion (Synchronized)	MT Practice	A-11	CD-ROM
Cardioverter Defibrillator Implantation	Proofreading & Editing Exercises	50	page 295
Carotid Duplex Scan	Proofreading & Editing Exercises	1	page 149
Catheterization and Ventriculography (Left Cardiac)	MT Practice	A-20	CD-ROM
Catheterization and Ventriculography (Left Heart) in Patient with Cardiomyopathy	Proofreading & Editing Exercises	21	page 209
Catheterization (Cardiac) with Pump Insertion and Pacemaker Wire Insertion	Proofreading & Editing Exercises	48	page 289
Catheterization (Cardiac) with Vein Graft and Left Internal Mammary Graft Angiography	Proofreading & Editing Exercises	43	page 275
Catheterization (Pediatric Diagnostic Cardiac)	MT Practice	A-41	CD-ROM

Report Topic	Section	Report #	Location
Echocardiogram with Doppler for Evaluation of Left Ventricular Function	Proofreading & Editing Exercises	23	page 213
Electrical Cardioversion	Proofreading & Editing Exercises	38	page 261
Electrophysiologic Study (Abnormal) for Patient with Severe Coronary Artery Disease	MT Practice	A-39	CD-ROM
Electrophysiologic Study (Abnormal) for Patient with Syncope	Proofreading & Editing Exercises	41	page 268
Electrophysiologic Study and Radiofrequency Catheter Ablation (Pediatric)	MT Practice	A-46	CD-ROM
Electrophysiologic Study for Patient with Ischemic Heart Disease	Proofreading & Editing Exercises	26	page 222
Electrophysiologic Study (Intracardiac) and Radiofrequency Catheter Ablation (Pediatric)	Proofreading & Editing Exercises	33	page 250
Electrophysiologic Study with Mapping and Isuprel Infusion	MT Practice	A-37	CD-ROM
Endoscopic Vein Harvest, Complex Valve Annuloplasty, Coronary Artery Bypass Graft, Radiofrequency Ablation and Transesophageal Echocardiography	MT Practice	A-43	CD-ROM
Exercise Stress Test (Pediatric)	MT Practice	A-15	CD-ROM
Exercise Stress Test Without Nuclear Injection	MT Practice	A-40	CD-ROM
Heart Murmur, Consultation for Patient with (Pediatric)	Proofreading & Editing Exercises	18	page 201
History and Physical Examination for Angina Pectoris	MT Practice	A-4	CD-ROM
History and Physical Examination for Atrial Fibrillation	Proofreading & Editing Exercises	11	page 176
History and Physical Examination for Chest Pain	Proofreading & Editing Exercises	4	page 156
History and Physical Examination for Shortness of Breath	Proofreading & Editing Exercises	9	page 170
Holter Monitor (24-Hour)	Proofreading & Editing Exercises	7	page 163
Holter Monitor (24-Hour)	MT Practice	A-16	CD-ROM
Imaging Study (Lower Extremity Graft)	Proofreading & Editing Exercises	35	page 255
Imaging Study (Right Groin)	Proofreading & Editing Exercises	36	page 257

Report Topic	Section	Report #	Location
Vein Graft, Cardiac Catheterization with Left Internal Mammary Graft Angiography and	Proofreading & Editing Exercises	43	page 275
Ventriculography and Catheterization (Left Cardiac)	MT Practice	A-20	CD-ROM
Ventriculography and Catheterization (Left Heart) in Patient with Cardiomyopathy	Proofreading & Editing Exercises	21	page 209

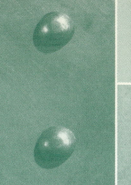

Terms Index

Page numbers in *italics* denote illustrations.